Telehealth

Editors

KATHRYN M. HARMES
ROBERT J. HEIZELMAN
JOEL J. HEIDELBAUGH

PRIMARY CARE:
CLINICS IN OFFICE PRACTICE

www.primarycare.theclinics.com

Consulting Editor
JOEL J. HEIDELBAUGH

December 2022 • Volume 49 • Number 4

ELSEVIER

1600 John F. Kennedy Boulevard • Suite 1800 • Philadelphia, Pennsylvania, 19103-2899

http://www.theclinics.com

PRIMARY CARE: CLINICS IN OFFICE PRACTICE Volume 49, Number 4
December 2022 ISSN 0095-4543, ISBN-13: 978-0-323-96157-8

Editor: Taylor Hayes
Developmental Editor: Jessica Cañaberal

Primary Care: Clinics in Office Practice (ISSN: 0095-4543) is published quarterly by Elsevier Inc., 360 Park Avenue South, New York, NY 10010-1710. Months of issue are March, June, September, and December. Periodicals postage paid at New York, NY and additional mailing offices. Subscription prices are $269.00 per year (US individuals), $672.00 (US institutions), $100.00 (US students), $312.00 (Canadian individuals), $696.00 (Canadian institutions), $100.00 (Canadian students), $368.00 (international individuals), $696.00 (international institutions), and $175.00 (international students). Foreign air speed delivery is included in all *Clinics* subscription prices. All prices are subject to change without notice. POSTMASTER: Send address changes to *Primary Care: Clinics in Office Practice*, Elsevier Periodicals Customer Service, 11830 Westline Industrial Drive, St. Louis, MO 63146. Customer Service Health Sciences Division, Subscription Customer Service, 3251 Riverport Lane, Maryland Heights, MO 63043. **Customer Service: 1-800-654-2452 (U.S. and Canada); 314-447-8871 (outside U.S. and Canada). Fax: 314-447-8029. E-mail: journalscustomerservice-usa@elsevier.com (for print support); journalsonlinesupport-usa@elsevier.com (for online support).**

Reprints. For copies of 100 or more, of articles in this publication, please contact the Commercial Reprints Department, Elsevier Inc., 360 Park Avenue South, New York, NY 10010-1710. Tel. 212-633-3874; Fax: 212-633-3820; E-mail: reprints@elsevier.com.

Primary Care: Clinics in Office Practice is covered in *MEDLINE/PubMed (Index Medicus)* and *EMBASE/Excerpta Medica, Current Contents/Clinical Medicine, and ISI/BIOMED.*

Contributors

CONSULTING EDITOR

JOEL J. HEIDELBAUGH, MD, FAAFP, FACG
Clinical Professor, Departments of Family Medicine and Urology, Director of Medical Student Education and Clerkship Director, Department of Family Medicine, University of Michigan Medical School, Ann Arbor, Michigan; Ypsilanti Health Center, Ypsilanti, Michigan

EDITORS

KATHRYN M. HARMES, MD, MHSA, FAAFP
Assistant Professor, Department of Family Medicine, University of Michigan Medical School, Ann Arbor, Michigan

ROBERT J. HEIZELMAN, MD
Clinical Assistant Professor, Department of Family Medicine, University of Michigan Medical School, Ann Arbor, Michigan

JOEL J. HEIDELBAUGH, MD, FAAFP, FACG
Clinical Professor, Departments of Family Medicine and Urology, Director of Medical Student Education and Clerkship Director, Department of Family Medicine, University of Michigan Medical School, Ann Arbor, Michigan; Ypsilanti Health Center, Ypsilanti, Michigan

AUTHORS

ERIC W. BEAN, DO, MBA, FACEP
Clinical Assistant Professor, Department of Emergency and Hospital Medicine, Lehigh Valley Health Network, Allentown, Pennsylvania

ALEKSANDR BELAKOVSKIY, MD
Assistant Professor, University of Michigan Medical School, Ann Arbor, Michigan

SHANDRA M. BROWN LEVEY, PhD
Department of Family Medicine, University of Colorado School of Medicine, Aurora, Colorado

ANDREA B. BUCHI, MD
Clinical Instructor, Department of Pediatrics, University of Michigan, Virtual Care Department, Ann Arbor, Michigan

STEPHANIE CALLAN, MA
University of Colorado Denver, Denver, Colorado

RAMON S. CANCINO, MD, MBA, MS, FAAFP
Department of Family & Community Medicine, Joe R & Teresa Lozano Long School of Medicine, UT Health San Antonio, San Antonio, Texas

VICTORIA CHESTNUT, DNP, MBA, RN
Lehigh Valley Health Network CARES Center, Allentown, Pennsylvania

GRANT M. GREENBERG, MD, MA, MHSA, FAAFP
Leonard Parker Pool Endowed Chair of Family Medicine, Lehigh Valley Health Network,
Associate Professor of Medical Education and Family Medicine, University of South
Florida Morsani College of Medicine, LVHN-One City Center, Allentown, Pennsylvania

KATHRYN M. HARMES, MD, MHSA, FAAFP
Clinical Associate Professor, Department of Family Medicine, University of Michigan
Medical School, Ann Arbor, Michigan

LAURA HEINRICH, MD
Assistant Professor and Assistant Residency Director, Department of Family Medicine,
University of Michigan, Primary Care Physician Lead, Virtual Care Department, University
of Michigan Health, Ann Arbor, Michigan

ROBERT J. HEIZELMAN, MD
Clinical Assistant Professor, Department of Family Medicine, The University of Michigan,
Ann Arbor, Michigan

ANITA K. HERNANDEZ, MD
Assistant Professor and Service Director of Family Mother Baby, Department of Family
Medicine, University of Michigan, Ann Arbor, Michigan

HEATHER HOLMSTROM, MD, FAAFP
University of Colorado Anschutz, Aurora, Colorado; UC Health Family Medicine-Boulder,
Boulder, Colorado

MOLLY HOSS, MD
Assistant Professor, Department of Family Medicine, University of Colorado Anschutz
Medical Campus, Aurora, Colorado

CHARISSE HUOT, MD, FAAFP
University of South Florida Morsani College of Medicine, University of South Florida/
Morton Plant Mease Family Medicine Residency, Dr. Joseph A. Eaddy Family Medicine
Research Center, Turley Family Health Center, Clearwater, Florida

JULIA C. JENKINS, MD, FAAFP
University of South Florida Morsani College of Medicine, University of South Florida/
Morton Plant Mease Family Medicine Residency, Dr. Joseph A. Eaddy Family Medicine
Research Center, Turley Family Health Center, Clearwater, Florida

TRACY JOHNS, PharmD, MSMS, BCACP
University of South Florida Morsani College of Medicine, University of South Florida/
Morton Plant Mease Family Medicine Residency, Dr. Joseph A. Eaddy Family Medicine
Research Center, Turley Family Health Center, Clearwater, Florida

ELIZABETH K. JONES, MD
Assistant Professor, University of Michigan Medical School, Ann Arbor, Michigan

MARISA KOSTIUK, PhD
Licensed Psychologist, Senior Instructor, University of Colorado, Westminster, Colorado

ERIK S. KRAMER, DO, MPH, Dipl. of ABOM
Department of Family Medicine, University of Colorado Anschutz, Aurora, Colorado

ROBERT KRUKLITIS, MD, PhD, MBA
Lehigh Valley Health Network CARES Center, Allentown, Pennsylvania

ANNA R. LAURIE, MD
Assistant Professor and Director of Population Health, Department of Family Medicine, University of Michigan, Ann Arbor, Michigan

DEBRA M. LANGLOIS, MD
Clinical Assistant Professor, Department of Pediatrics, University of Michigan, Canton, Michigan

COREY LYON, DO
Associate Professor, Associate Vice Chair for Clinical Affairs Department of Family Medicine, University of Colorado School of Medicine, Aurora, Colorado

MATTHEW B. MACKWOOD, MD, MPH
Department of Community and Family Medicine, Geisel School of Medicine, Dartmouth, Hanover, New Hampshire

NAOMI MALAM, MD, MSPH
Assistant Professor, Department of Family Medicine, University of Colorado Anschutz Medical Campus, Aurora, Colorado

MATTHEW MILLER, DO, MBA
Cleveland Clinic, Cleveland, Ohio

AMEET S. NAGPAL, MD, MS, MEd, MBA
Department of Orthopaedics and Physical Medicine, Medical University of South Carolina, Charleston, South Carolina

REBECCA NORTHWAY, MD
Clinical Assistant Professor, Departments of Pediatrics and Internal Medicine, University of Michigan, Canton, Michigan

NADINE OPSTBAUM, MBA
Lehigh Valley Health Network CARES Center, Allentown, Pennsylvania

CHRISTINA S. PALMER, MD
Department of Family Medicine, University of Colorado School of Medicine

REBECCA M. RICHEY, PsyD
University of Colorado, Denver, Colorado

JULIA SHAVER, MD
Primary Care Innovations Director, Kaiser Santa Rosa Family Medicine Residency, Kaiser Permanente Northern California, Santa Rosa, California; Volunteer Clinical Faculty, Department of Family and Community Medicine, University of California San Francisco, California

STEVEN SHINE, BSE
Lehigh Valley Health Network CARES Center, Allentown, Pennsylvania

ALISON SHMERLING, MD, MPH
Assistant Clinical Professor, Department of Family Medicine, University of Colorado Anschutz Medical Campus, Aurora, Colorado

ELIZABETH W. STATON, MSTC
Senior Instructor, Department of Family Medicine, University of Colorado Anschutz Medical Campus, Aurora, Colorado

JENNIFER STEPHENS, DO, MBA, FACP
Chief Value and Ambulatory Care Officer, Lehigh Valley Health Network, Chief Medical Officer, Lehigh Valley Physicians Group, Assistant Professor of Medical Education and Medicine, University of South Florida Morsani College of Medicine, Assistant Clinical Professor, Philadelphia College of Osteopathic Medicine, LVHN-One City Center, Allentown, Pennsylvania

LAUREN WOODWARD TOLLE, PhD
Department of Family Medicine, University of Colorado School of Medicine, Aurora, Colorado

LORRAINE VALERIANO, BSN, CNRN, CHC
Lehigh Valley Health Network CARES Center, Allentown, Pennsylvania

JILL VANWYK, MD
University of Colorado Anschutz, Aurora, Colorado; UC Health Family Medicine-Boulder, Boulder, Colorado

JOYCE YUEN, DO
Department of Family & Community Medicine, Joe R & Teresa Lozano Long School of Medicine, UT Health San Antonio, San Antonio, Texas

AIMEE R. ZISNER, PhD, MSc
Department of Family Medicine, University of Colorado School of Medicine, Aurora, Colorado

Contents

> Telemedicine was underused and understudied until the COVID-19 pandemic, during which reduced regulations and increased payment parity facilitated a rapid increase in telemedicine consultation. Telemedicine literature to date suggests that it holds benefits for patients and health care providers, may result in outcomes not inferior to in-person care, and has cost-saving implications. Future research should investigate which conditions are best suited to assess and treat via telemedicine (including physical exam elements), what techniques improve telemedicine communication, how to help patients equitably access telemedicine, and how to best educate the future health care workforce.

> Asynchronous telehealth provides a viable option for improving access in a convenient and timely manner to patients seeking care as well as for physicians seeking subspecialty consultation. Access to technology, clear guidelines, standards, and expectations is required for this innovation to function well. Limitations in access due to patient and technology factors is an area that requires attention. Positive impact on access and quality has been demonstrated. Rapid development continues and was enhanced with the Sars-CoV-2 pandemic.

> Remote patient monitoring programs collect and analyze a variety of health-related data to detect clinical deterioration with the goal of early intervention. There are many program designs with various deployed devices, monitoring schemes, and escalation protocols. Although several factors are considered, the disease state plays a foundational role when designing a specific program. Remote patient monitoring is used both in chronic disease states and patients with acute self-limited conditions. These programs use health-related data to identify early deterioration and then successfully intervene to improve clinical outcomes and decrease costs of care.

Telehealth programs existed in many subspecialities before the COVID-19 pandemic, and the public health event motivated many subspecialties to reflect on how current technologies could be leveraged to benefit patient outcomes and increase health-care access. This article reviews the history and current state of telehealth access in many areas of subspecialty care. Primary care physicians (PCPs) may be unaware of the telehealth services and options local subspecialists offer. To best serve patients, PCPs could partner with subspecialists to develop processes to link patients to the right subspecialist at the right time and in the right visit type.

As telehealth continues to evolve, there is a subsequent need to develop efficient and effective teaching models in this realm. Primary care is well positioned to teach telehealth because of the breadth of medical conditions treated. It is crucial that learners and medical educators are prepared for learning and educating in this growing paradigm. This article offers an organized approach to education in telehealth that includes preparation, observation, assessment, and feedback.

This article discusses the use of telehealth in the role of pediatric health care. Management of common pediatric complaints and concerns are discussed in the context of a virtual setting. Benefits, as well as limitations and challenges, and the future of telehealth within the care of pediatric patient are reviewed.

Recent rapid expansion of telemedicine services has included delivery of those services to adolescents and young adults. Telemedicine can be used to provide a wide array of health services to adolescent and young adult (AYA) including the treatment of mental health and substance use disorders, gender-affirming services, contraception, acute care, and health education. Special attention to minor consent laws which vary by state and country should help inform the health system and practice decisions for patient portal access, delivery of confidential care, and care for which the consent of a guardian or parent is required. For AYA with limited transportation options or who are geographically distant from specialty care, telemedicine helps expand access to those services.

During the COVID-19 pandemic, providers and patients explored the use of telehealth on a wide and rapid scale. Reflecting on how prenatal providers and pregnant patients used telehealth during the pandemic and afterward, we review existing and new lessons learned from the pandemic. This article summarizes international and national guidelines on prenatal care, presents practice examples on how telehealth and remote patient monitoring were used during the COVID-19 pandemic, and offers lessons learned and suggestions for future care.

The article summarizes the current state of hypertension management via telehealth. Included is information about diagnosis and management of hypertension in general, the role of telehealth regarding hypertension management, a description of self-measurement blood pressure monitoring, billing and coding for hypertension management via telehealth, and a discussion of hypertension quality metrics.

The care of patients with diabetes is complex and longitudinal. Improved management of diabetic risk factors can decrease long-term complications such as cardiovascular disease, renal failure, vision impairment, and amputation. A variety of telehealth options are available which may improve patient access to needed care as well as a provider understanding of the challenges for an individual patient. Health care teams must be thoughtful about how best to incorporate telehealth into the care of patients with diabetes.

The COVID-19 pandemic has highlighted the urgent need for behavioral health care services. A substantial portion of mental health care transitioned to virtual care during the COVID-19 pandemic, remains virtual today, and will continue that way in the future. Mental health needs continue to grow, and there has been growing evidence showing the efficacy of virtual health for behavioral health conditions at the system, provider, and patient level. There is also a growing understanding of the barriers and challenges to virtual behavioral health care.

Telehealth is commonly used in the care of geriatric patients; however, it requires special considerations for effective implementation. Although available evidence suggests that this model of care is useful and feasible, interventions should be carefully designed with the unique needs of geriatric patients in mind. Further, more research is needed to determine the most effective telehealth interventions in this population, which will assist in determining cost-effectiveness and reimbursement policies.

Urgent care as a distinct clinical care entity began in the 1970s to treat low-acuity conditions. Virtual urgent care (VUC) can be provided by the primary care physician (PCP) or home health system of the patient, and many commercial direct-to-consumer (DTC) companies have emerged to provide this service. Quality of care continues to be evaluated, but some studies suggest that DTC providers prescribe antibiotics at a higher rate than PCPs. VUC has been proposed to improve equity and access to care, but early evidence is mixed. New utilization owing to convenience may lead to overall higher health care costs.

PRIMARY CARE:
CLINICS IN OFFICE PRACTICE

SERIES OF RELATED INTEREST

Medical Clinics (http://www.medical.theclinics.com)
Physician Assistant Clinics (https://www.physicianassistant.theclinics.com)

THE CLINICS ARE AVAILABLE ONLINE!
Access your subscription at:
www.theclinics.com

PRIMARY CARE:
CLINICS IN OFFICE PRACTICE

Foreword
"Is This Legit?"

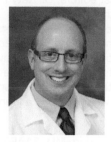

Joel J. Heidelbaugh, MD, FAAFP, FACG
Consulting Editor

One of the most exciting aspects of my career in academic family medicine is that it is always evolving, always driving innovation, and clinicians need to embrace change to stay at the top of our game and provide the best possible care for patients. Before the COVID-19 pandemic, I remember hearing about how our practices would be taking a quantum leap forward by seeing patients via a virtual platform. Admittedly, I was initially lost on this notion. A member of our institutional leadership had spoken to our department about this new idea of "video visits," and how he had engaged with a patient for a postoperative visit when the patient was in a deer blind in the woods. The patient was able to show the surgeon his healing wounds; he answered some questions about his postoperative state, and the visit concluded. Hearing this story for the first time stirred many questions in my mind: *"is this legit?," "wait a minute—how did he pull that off without doing a physical examination?,"* and *"can we really bill for this?."*

The reality is that we have proven that we can provide excellent care of our patients via a virtual platform within a short period of time, borne out of necessity during the pandemic. Psychiatric health care and counseling have thrived in this arena, offering services at unconventional hours, and I suspect they will continue to do so. Many routine follow-up visits have been successfully conducted, and we have created another avenue through which patients can obtain health care. The virtual medium can also reduce barriers to care impacted by social determinants, improve satisfaction with patient care, decrease health care costs, and augment outcomes.

This issue of *Primary Care: Clinics in Office Practice* dedicated to telehealth is a landmark with respect to its scope and expert guidance on how to optimize telehealth services across the spectrum of health care. The article that highlights applications of remote patient monitoring provides a paradigm for chronic disease management through asynchronous care and dovetails well with the articles on the interface between telehealth and hypertension and diabetes management. Additional articles

Prim Care Clin Office Pract 49 (2022) xiii–xiv
https://doi.org/10.1016/j.pop.2022.07.004
0095-4543/22/© 2022 Published by Elsevier Inc.

detail provisions for telehealth and prenatal care, pediatrics and adolescent medicine, geriatrics, urgent care, and subspecialty care. Last, an article dedicated to how we can best integrate virtual care in medical education serves as an integral paradigm upon which to build a novel teaching model.

I would like to acknowledge the incredible dedication and contributions to this issue of *Primary Care: Clinics in Office Practice* from my coguest editors, Dr Katy Harmes and Dr Robert Heizelman. As mutual colleagues in the Department of Family Medicine at the University of Michigan, it is a privilege to watch their leadership in our department and institution drive telehealth innovations forward as we advance population health initiatives. I am indebted to our many expert authors, who have provided substantial contributions via their articles. I suspect that this will be the first of many collections of publications on various aspects of telehealth, and I hope that our readers will find this to be one of many elements upon which to build a foundation of new knowledge and skills in daily practice.

Joel J. Heidelbaugh, MD, FAAFP, FACG
Departments of Family Medicine and Urology
Department of Family Medicine
University of Michigan Medical School
Ann Arbor, MI, USA

Ypsilanti Health Center
200 Arnet Suite 200
Ypsilanti, MI 48198, USA

E-mail address:
jheidel@umich.edu

Preface

The Doctor Is Online: The New Virtual Landscape of Health Care

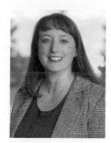
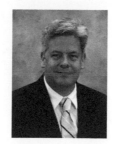

Kathryn M. Harmes, MD, MHSA, FAAFP   Robert J. Heizelman, MD
Editors

Telehealth existed prior to the COVID-19 pandemic, but the sudden decrease in availability of face-to-face care resulted in rapid expansion of virtual technologies as patients and caregivers found alternative means to connect to each other.[1,2] The expansion of telehealth was further facilitated by relaxation of billing rules under the Public Health Emergency determination.[3] As primary care physicians, specialists, and direct-to-consumer companies expand telehealth offerings evidence on the quality, safety, cost-effectiveness, and equity of care continues to emerge but lags implementation in many areas.

In the post-COVID environment, we can expect telehealth to remain an established method of health care delivery. Video technology is available in the palm of the hand and in the functionality of electronic medical record. Patients will continue to demand increased convenience with less cost. Health care providers are challenged to adjust to this new reality, without the support of training or experience or solid evidence in many cases.

This issue seeks to provide primary care physicians with tools to address this challenge. Use of telehealth is explored in specific populations including pediatrics, adolescents, geriatrics, and prenatal care. Application of telehealth in the management of hypertension, diabetes, and behavioral care is discussed. Telehealth is examined in environments our patients access outside of primary care such as specialty and urgent care. Specific technologies, including remote patient monitoring and asynchronous care, are demonstrated. One article addresses the role of virtual care in medical education, to prepare our future physicians to use the technology effectively.

Evidence supporting the use of telehealth is included where available but we recognize that this is an emerging field and expert opinion is included where evidence is

Prim Care Clin Office Pract 49 (2022) xv–xvi
https://doi.org/10.1016/j.pop.2022.07.003
0095-4543/22/© 2022 Published by Elsevier Inc.

unavailable. We greatly appreciate the efforts of all of our authors, who have been responding to recurrent COVID surges while contributing to this issue.

Kathryn M. Harmes, MD, MHSA, FAAFP
University of Michigan Medical School
300 North Ingalls Street, NI4C06
Ann Arbor, MI 48109-5435, USA

Robert J. Heizelman, MD
University of Michigan Medical School
300 North Ingalls Street, NI4C06
Ann Arbor, MI 48109-5435, USA

E-mail addresses:
jordankm@umich.edu (K.M. Harmes)
roheizel@umich.edu (R.J. Heizelman)

REFERENCES

1. Koonin LM, Hoots B, Tsang CA, et al. Trends in the use of telehealth during the emergency of the COVID-19 pandemic—United States, January–March 2020. MMWR Morb Mortal Wkly Rep 2020;69:1595–9.
2. The Chartis Group. Telehealth Adoption Tracker 2021. Available at: https://reports.chartis.com/telehealth_trends_and_implications-2021/. Accessed April 13, 2022.
3. US Department of Health and Human Services. Public Health Emergency. Updated April 2021. Available at: https://www.phe.gov/emergency/news/healthactions/phe/Pages/COVID-15April2021.aspx. Accessed April 13, 2022.

The State of Telehealth Before and After the COVID-19 Pandemic

Julia Shaver, MD*

KEYWORDS

- Telemedicine • Telehealth • COVID-19 • Health care outcomes • Access
- Health equity • Education

KEY POINTS

- Telemedicine health care has grown in the United States since the beginning of the COVID-19 pandemic and will remain an integral part of medical care.
- Telemedicine is well received by many patients and health care providers but remains more accessible to certain groups of patients than others.
- Telemedicine care can be equivalent to in-person care for certain acute and chronic conditions. The telemedicine physical examination should be further studied for how it may contribute to patient assessment.
- Future clinicians and all levels of learners within health care will require more specific training on how to logistically manage telemedicine technology and how to clinically navigate a remote consultation.

INTRODUCTION

The "house call" from doctors is surging in the United States, and instead of ringing the doorbell, your doctor is pinging your smartphone. Telemedicine, or receiving one's medical care remotely via synchronous, asynchronous, or store-and-forward technology, had been on a steady increase for the last decade, but the overall growth had remained slow until March 6, 2020. In response to the SARS-CoV-2 pandemic crisis, the US Congress toppled a multitude of telemedicine regulations, and telemedicine expanded rapidly. Although the acute pandemic crisis may be entering its long tail, telemedicine will remain a permanent fixture in routine American health care. How will this serve us as practitioners and patrons of medicine? The experiences of the last several years can help us forge our path forward into a future with virtual health care.

Kaiser Permanente Northern California, Santa Rosa, CA, USA
* 401 Bicentennial Way, Santa Rosa, CA 95403.
E-mail address: Julia.m.shaver@kp.org

Prim Care Clin Office Pract 49 (2022) 517–530
https://doi.org/10.1016/j.pop.2022.04.002
primarycare.theclinics.com

Definitions of Telemedicine and Telehealth

The definitions of these two terms depend upon whom you ask and what you read, as there are currently more than one hundred different peer-reviewed definitions.[1] A general consensus shared by most is that telemedicine refers to providing clinical services (either in real time or asynchronously) between patient and clinician and/or between clinician and clinician when the two parties are physically remote from one another using some form of information-communication technology. The term telehealth is a larger umbrella term encompassing other remote health-related services, such as administration, continuing medical education, and/or provider training.

TELEMEDICINE IN THE UNITED STATES BEFORE MARCH 2020

Before March 2020, telemedicine use in the United States was on a steadily increasing trajectory, but its absolute integration remained low, and the logistics were complex.[2,3] Patients and providers who desired to use it navigated inconsistent and often inadequate reimbursement for services, restrictions on where each party must be located and what sort of technology interface they must use, and privacy regulations that necessitated costly investments in secure telecommunication technology. Providers were (and often still are even in a postpandemic landscape) limited from treating traveling patients by interstate licensing restrictions, and juggled miscellaneous rules about prescriptions, types of visits, and types of patients that were or were not acceptable for telemedicine.[4] Despite these hurdles, 76% of US hospital systems used some form of telemedicine as of 2018, with radiology, psychiatry, and cardiology noted as the highest users of the modality.[5] Systems factors, such as technology capability of the electronic medical record and other characteristics driven by reimbursement policies (such as rural location), influenced which hospitals or clinics were more likely to offer telehealth,[6,7] further limiting which patients had the option of using this service.

Of the patients who were able to access telemedicine before March 2020, their overall impressions were positive.[8–13] In a systematic review on the topic, the most frequently cited factors associated with patient telehealth satisfaction included improved outcomes (defined a variety of ways owing to heterogeneity of the 44 included studies), preferred modality over face-to-face visits, ease of use, low cost, improved communication, and elimination of travel time.[9] Patients also expressed some concerns about telemedicine, such as data security.[14] The telemedicine appointments assessed in these studies were almost entirely videoconferencing rather than telephone-only owing to reimbursement restrictions on the latter.

Clinicians had a more variable opinion of telemedicine, perhaps driven by inexperienceas most were not using it before the pandemicand those who did use it still conducted most of their visits in person. About half of clinicians surveyed in one setting (respondents largely consisting of psychiatry providers) who were actively using both telehealth and office visits in their practices were concerned that the personal connection through telehealth was inferior to office visits.[11] Approximately one-third of those clinicians also stated that the overall quality of the visit was better in person. Family medicine providers (N = 1630) surveyed about the reasons behind their nonuse of telehealth were more likely than current users to feel it was an inefficient use of their time, and to express concerns about the overall quality of care and the liability potential. Nonusers were also more likely to cite lack of training, equipment costs, liability concerns, and inadequate reimbursement as barriers to telehealth.[15]

COVID-19 DRIVES TELEHEALTH EXPANSION AND GIVES NEW INSIGHTS ON PATIENT AND PROVIDER USE

The widespread recognition of SARS-CoV-2 in the United States by March 2020 upended many of the prior barriers to telemedicine. Patients who would have had in-person office visits for their needs were isolating, quarantining, sheltering under health orders, or fearful to venture out. In early March 2020, Congress made major alterations to Medicare restrictions on where telemedicine must originate, what would be reimbursed, and what platforms could be used (**Table 1**). This paved the way for similar relaxations on interstate practice and privacy regulations, and reimbursements for telemedicine improved dramatically. State and private payors promptly followed Medicare's lead in a collective effort to keep health care channels open and practices solvent.[2]

In response, practices greatly expanded telemedicine services during the long months of shelter in place and recurrent surges of COVID-19 infections, and patient use of telehealth services blossomed. A national study including 36 million working-age individuals with private insurance claims data showed that telemedicine encounters increased 766% in the first 3 months of the pandemic, from 0.3% of all

Table 1
Comparison of Centers for Medicare & Medicaid Services telehealth regulations before and after March 2020

Before March 2020	After CARES Act and CMS 1135 Waiver
Who can perform and receive telehealth	
Only certain licensed providers	Any type of clinician can bill for Medicare services
Patients and providers who have a preexisting relationship	No preexisting relationship will be required
Where can telehealth be done	
Only at prespecified sites (ie, designated rural areas, certain medical facilities)	Telehealth may originate and be conducted from any site, including patient's home
Physicians must conduct telehealth from their place of practice	Physicians may conduct telehealth from home
Telehealth may not cross state lines	Telehealth can now be provided to patient in another state (state-specific restrictions may still apply)
What must be used for telehealth visits	
Must be audio-visual (ie, video technology)	Audio-visual OR audio-only are allowed
Only approved technology platforms	Expanded approved platforms, including FaceTime, Skype, and Zoom
How is telehealth reimbursed	
Medicare coinsurance and deductibles apply to telehealth visits	Providers may waive cost-sharing for telehealth paid for by federal programs
Reimbursements for telehealth services is lower than for in-person services	All telehealth visits, including audio-only, will be reimbursed as if the service was furnished in person

Data from CARES Act AMA Covid-19 Fact Sheet (https://www.ama-assn.org/delivering-care/public-health/cares-act-ama-covid-19-pandemic-telehealth-fact-sheet) and Medicare Telemedicine Healthcare Provider Fact Sheet (https://www.cms.gov/newsroom/fact-sheets/medicare-telemedicine-health-care-provider-fact-sheet). Accessed 2/2/2022.

interactions in March to June 2019, to 23.6% of all interactions in the same period.[16] This is in line with research by the Doximity online medical networking service, which counts 1.8 million physicians (about 80% of the US physician workforce) among its membership, estimating with private claims data that approximately 20% of all US health care visits in 2020 were conducted by telemedicine.[17] However, even as telemedicine skyrocketed, medical care in general across the United States showed a sharp decline that could not be made whole despite best efforts. One estimate using claims data from 16.7 million Medicare Advantage and commercial insurance patients estimated that total outpatient visits plummeted by 30% of usual volume between January and June 2020, and that telemedicine only compensated for about two-thirds of this loss.[18] Physicians across the nation were severely impacted between reduction in overall visit volume, increased spending on personal protective equipment, and pervasive staffing challenges. Eighty percent of physicians surveyed by the American Medical Association reported a persistent reduction in income (average reported decrease of 32%) at 5 months into the pandemic.[19]

Even as isolation precautions have relaxed and shelter-in-place orders are past, telehealth is showing some staying power. FAIRHealth,[20] which manages a large national database of both private and Medicare claims data, shows that although in-person care is still chosen most of the time, the overall percentage of telehealth claims has ballooned from 0.1% in 2019 to hover just around 5% at the close of 2021 (**Fig. 1**).

DISCUSSION: TELEMEDICINE DURING AND AFTER COVID-19
Who Is Using Telemedicine Now?

Although disappearing regulations have somewhat leveled the playing field for all to participate, there are still various factors that predict which physicians and which patients are more likely to engage in telemedicine. What we know about physicians accessing telemedicine comes from studies of large academic practices, claims data from commercial insurance, and research from Doximity.

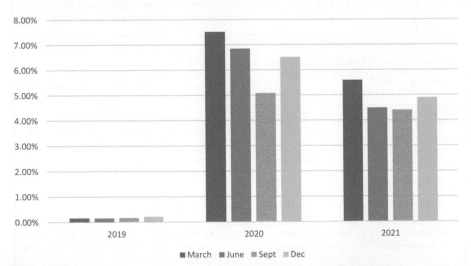

Fig. 1. Telehealth claims (as a percentage of all claims) in the United States from 2019 to 2021, based on FAIRHealth reported claims data, which includes participating Medicare and private insurance plans. (*Data from* FAIRHealth Monthly Telehealth Regional Tracker. https://www.fairhealth.org/states-by-the-numbers/telehealth. Accessed 12/10/2021.)

According to available data, the number of physicians reporting telemedicine as an active skill has doubled as of 2020, from 20% to just less than 40% of the Doximity survey.[17] A physician most likely to be practicing telehealth today treats patients who have chronic diseases, such as in endocrinology, gastroenterology, rheumatology, nephrology, cardiology, and psychiatry, whereas physicians in dermatology, orthopedic surgery, or optometry are least likely to report telemedicine use (note: these references did not distinguish between subspecialists who treat chronic disease and primary care physicians who may treat the same conditions).[17,18,21] Telemedicine practitioners tend to identify as female more often than male and are between 40 and 60 years of age.[17] They live predominantly in large metropolitan areas or on the East Coast.[17,18] The clinician demographics are likely influenced by the inherent demographics of the high-telemedicine specialties.

As telehealth rapidly evolves, it is important to note what has changed (and what has not) now that insurance type, physical location, and technology platform should present fewer barriers for all to use telemedicine. Historically, it has been challenging to describe the typical "telemedicine user," because telemedicine use was such a small proportion of care before the pandemic. What has been reported about the demographics of telemedicine users before 2020 reflects what would be expected of those select patients that either were granted access (eg, large academic centers, Veterans Administration health system, integrated health systems) or purchased access (eg, through direct-to-consumer telemedicine services). In contrast, some patients who might be expected to frequently use telemedicine (including those who live far away from in-person care, such as large areas in the middle of the United States) were often effectively excluded owing to lower rates of household internet access. Others who suffered from the digital divide included households of lower socioeconomic status and patients with disabilities.[22]

With the advent of the pandemic in 2020, reimbursable telemedicine services expanded to include telephone-only visits and removed geographic barriers and platform restrictions. Interestingly, this has not addressed the inequities in telemedicine use as much as one might predict. Studies inclusive of March to August 2020, which examined demographics of new telemedicine users, show a surprisingly similar picture to the prepandemic period: patients who use telemedicine still tend to be white, younger, wealthier, and more urban-dwelling than non-telemedicine-using peers.[16,23–26] This demographic discrepancy becomes even more apparent when examining video telemedicine users compared with telephone (audio-only) users.[23,24,26] Although this picture of the typical telemedicine user may reflect the larger troubling patterns of inequitable access to medical care in general in our country, these data should still guide us as we move into a more telemedicine-dependent future. Our most vulnerable, marginalized, and chronically ill patients will need additional attention and funding dollars to understand all their barriers (digital and otherwise) to this type of care that we hope could address their care gaps, and to prevent telemedicine from becoming yet another wedge to widen medical disparities in our country.

Despite the observed differences in utilization, telemedicine visits did globally increase for all types of patients compared with rates in 2019 and prior, especially among those with chronic illnesses.[17] Perceptions of telemedicine care from this much larger sample of users continue to be positive overall whether they are new to telemedicine or experienced. One survey of 800 patients at Penn Medicine in the first half of 2020 reported that 67% of respondents considered their video or telephone visit "as good or better" than a standard in-person visit.[27] A similar survey of 1011 University of Michigan Medicine patients in early 2020 showed similar degrees of high satisfaction between first-time users and repeat patient users of telemedicine.[28] In addition, although telemedicine use varies significantly based on certain demographics (as described above) because of either preference or barriers, those who use it across different demographics can have a similar experience. A nationally representative sample of US households (N = 3454) surveyed on telemedicine use during the pandemic affirmed that telemedicine use differed significantly based on race, household income, insurance status, and presence of high-speed internet (in keeping with the literature cited above), but that those who did use telemedicine even in lower-income households or non-white households seemed equally satisfied with their experience.[29]

What Do We Know About Conditions that Are Evaluated by Telemedicine?

In the literature to date, telemedicine is most often evaluated by examining patient acceptance of care using technology, patient and clinician satisfaction with the visit, and patient perception of care they received. Studies examining patient-oriented health outcomes or economic impact on individuals and systems are less common and are needed to delineate how telemedicine can be best used for future medical care.

Before the COVID-19 pandemic, research on telemedicine health care outcomes had some inherent challenges. Patients using telemedicine were a self-selected audience with the inherent differences that accompany this, and telemedicine is a broad category that encompasses many different intervention types ranging from simple telephone encounters to highly intensive encounters involving facilitators or digital examination equipment, such as stethoscopes or otoscopes able to transmit audiovisual information to a remote provider. Likewise, it is challenging to compare outcomes between telemedicine and face-to-face care in a prepandemic world where clinicians might prioritize in-person encounters for more high-risk or medically complex individuals when there is no limitation or disincentive for doing so.

Despite these challenges, there is now more literature to support telemedicine as a viable alternative to in-person care in certain situations. One of the more comprehensive looks at this topic was a systematic review of telemedicine practice in primary care before the pandemic, including 81 studies conducted both domestically and abroad.[30] The results from this study have been supplemented by other publications conducted during the pandemic, and general conclusions about patient outcomes for different categories of careare summarized below.

Acute care using telemedicine

Telemedicine has been studied in various acute conditions as compared with usual care, including uncomplicated cystitis, upper respiratory tract infections (URI), pharyngitis, and low-back pain. Results of these studies are heterogenous. Some suggest that telemedicine care for conditions such as URI and low-back pain can result in similar or improved clinical outcomes for patients, with "clinical outcomes" usually defined narrowly as a single categorical item (such as appropriate vs inappropriate use of antibiotics for a given diagnosis). In a nurse-administered telephone or a Web-based protocol for URI and sinusitis treatment, overall antibiotic administration with telemedicine for viral URI was less than usual care, and first-line antibiotics were more often prescribed for cases of sinusitis meeting clinical criteria.[31,32] In an evaluation of care administered by Teladoc, a direct-to-consumer telemedicine consultation service, telemedicine consultations did *not* order imaging for low-back pain (appropriately so) at about the same rate as in-person evaluations.[33]

Other studies in direct-to-consumer telemedicine differ, suggesting that patients who received telemedicine may be more likely to receive inappropriate antibiotics than when seen in face-to-face care[33–35] and are less likely to receive an appropriate rapid strep test for evaluation of pharyngitis.[33] The variations in medication use and diagnostic testing seen in these studies may be explained by the context of a direct-to-consumer telemedicine encounter. The typical model for direct-to-consumer telemedicine is a single encounter between a clinician and patient who have no preceding relationship, and the clinician is often limited by lack of on-site testing, no means to bring patient in for a face-to-face examination, and little way to ensure the patient will access follow-up care if they get worse. Telemedicine outcomes may look different when delivered within a context where physicians and patients know one another, a consistent medical record is available, on-site testing may be achievable, and there is more readily accessible follow-up care. An observational study in this type of setting (a large integrated health system) analyzed more than 1 million visits: telephone, video, and office visits, for any type of initial concern (excluding routine physical examination) during a 2-year period. Patients initiated scheduling of the visit modality themselves via a Web-based scheduling portal. The investigators found that rates of overall prescribing of medication or imaging (across all diagnoses as well as a subanalysis of visits only for URI symptoms) were actually lower for telemedicine (telephone or video) as opposed to in-person care, and that the need for emergency department (ED) or hospital visit within 7 days following the index visit did not differ between telemedicine and in person.[36] This suggests that clinicians using telemedicine may be less likely to overprescribe or overuse testing as a precautionary measure when they have some prior knowledge of the patient and when they feel confident that follow-up care is available should things get worse.

This study also demonstrates that when examined in a very large sample and over a broad array of diagnoses, assessment and treatment via telemedicine seem no more likely to result in acute decompensation requiring emergency room services or hospitalization than traditional in-person care. However, emergency and hospital care is an uncommon outcome to begin with; in this study, overall rates of ER visits within a week of index visits were approximately 1% across all visit types, and hospitalizations were less than 0.5%. Future studies may do well to see if this conclusion holds true when telemedicine care is used for specific diagnoses (dizziness, abdominal pain, dyspnea) that may be more challenging to assess, or for different types of telemedicine users that may have communication barriers.

For acute skin concerns, tele-dermatology is already used in multiple countries for routine dermatologic management, to consult on patients in remote locales, or for medical support in nursing homes or home care settings.[37] However, most studies to this point have not examined a specific comparison with usual (in-person) consultation. Tele-dermatology may serve an intuitive role as a follow-up method once a diagnosis has been established, to triage whether an in-person consultation is needed, or to guide primary physicians on the best next steps in management for routine conditions.

Chronic care using telemedicine
Telemedicine has been studied for many chronic conditions, such as asthma, chronic obstructive pulmonary disease (COPD), depression, diabetes, hypertension, hyperlipidemia, and heart failure. Some of the most robust evidence for improved patient outcomes with telemedicine care comes from pharmacist-based telemedicine interventions. A systematic review of 34 studies looking at chronic disease management using pharmacist-delivered telemedicine care protocols examined outcomes for different conditions (hypertension, diabetes, anticoagulation, depression, hyperlipidemia, asthma, heart failure, HIV, posttraumatic stress disorder, chronic kidney

disease, stroke, COPD, and smoking cessation).[38] The investigators noted the heterogeneity of studies and for this reason did not perform a data synthesis to quantify collective results and instead performed a narrative review. Most included studies (N = 25) examined telephone-only interventions as opposed to more technology-intensive ones, and studies were included in the final review if they used a comparison (ie, face-to-face, usual care, or no intervention) and if they evaluated as outcomes either chronic disease management (ie, achievement of laboratory values specific to therapeutic goals), patient self-management (ie, self-monitoring blood pressure or demonstration of inhaler use), or adherence (ie, patient self-report or pharmacy records showing medication fills). Results showed good success for telemedicine interventions, with 23 out of 34 studies logging positive improvements in disease management, self-management, or adherence measures. Another 10 studies reported neutral outcomes (noninferior to the comparison), and only one study concluded any sort of negative outcome for the telemedicine group. A scheduled model of care, described as pharmacists delivering telemedicine interventions to patients at predetermined times, was the most common and the most successful delivery system for improved outcomes as opposed to a responsive/reactive model (pharmacist reaching out to patient when being prompted to do so by a health system alert). Similar benefits of pharmacist-led virtual care have been documented as health systems rapidly transitioned chronic disease care to virtual visits during the pandemic.[39]

One notable aspect of this systemic review is the increased success of scheduled telemedicine care as opposed to a more responsive/reactive model, affirming that a high degree of reinforcement and support is beneficial for chronic disease management in general whether in person or otherwise. Shifting some of this care to telemedicine could conceivably lower overall system costs through reduced overhead and possibly improved patient outcomes (if evidence cited above proves accurate) but would likely require upfront investment in clinicians or other personnel to support the consistent, high-frequency visits. The overall impact on physician and practice revenue is also unclear, as reimbursement for telemedicine may become less favorable when the pandemic wanes.

Other small studies show some benefit of telemedicine for other chronic conditions. One study demonstrates that telemedicine intervention delivered over an extended period (ie, 24 months) can be as successful as in-person care for weight loss of primary care patients, with either telemedicine or in-person treatment groups achieving equivalent weight loss and more so than the "no-treatment" arm.[40] Telemedicine also shows some promise with management of chronic musculoskeletal pain; patients who participate in a 12-month telemedicine intervention with algorithmic guide to pharmacologic management had improved pain scores at 1 year as compared with usual care.[41]

Despite the promise of evidence above, conclusions about telemedicine effectiveness overall can be difficult to determine, as the types and intensity of interventions vary drastically from study to study. In the case of asthma care, for example, one frequently cited telemedicine study entitled "Telemedicine is as effective as in-person visits for patients with asthma" concludes that children in the telemedicine group and children in an in-person visit group had similar degrees of asthma control over a 6-month study period.[42] However, the intervention described in the article is a highly intensive "Remote Presence Solution" involving a digital stethoscope and otoscope and a high-resolution camera situated at the patient's home site. Therefore, broad conclusions about equivalency of care must be interpreted in the context of the intervention being delivered (and whether it is feasible in most practices) as well as the outcome of interest, all of which tend to be variable across telemedicine literature. A more recent narrative review on the topic of asthma care via telemedicine looked at a variety of interventions ranging from telephone-only follow-ups to the Remote Presence Solution described above, and concluded that data remain limited for clinical outcomes on this condition.[43] In addition, many studies in this review that used a telemedicine intervention combined it with a school-based care program, making it difficult to conclude what effects (if any) might be due to the telemedicine itself.

Similar challenges in drawing firm conclusions have been noted in a recent umbrella review of systematic reviews regarding telemedicine interventions for diabetes care, cholesterol, and hypertension.[44] Although the investigators concluded that telemedicine may improve outcomes for patients with diabetes and there are trends favoring certain subgroups in other conditions, the overall quality of the current evidence is low or very low because of potential bias in study design, heterogeneity in subgroups, imprecision of results or small effect sizes (due to small sample sizes), publication bias, and underreporting of relevant information, such as the treatment of dropout or missing data. Larger, more robust studies that address specific questions on clinical outcomes of telemedicine-supported chronic disease care as pandemic-era data come to publication are eagerly awaited.

Impacts on systems and resource utilization

Using telemedicine for select cases of both acute and chronic disease management may decrease the need for some routine face-to-face visits. In addition, there is interest in whether early triage and intervention for patient concerns via telemedicine could decrease face-to-face visits in urgent care and ED settings. A study by Reed and colleagues[36] showed that over a very large sample of appointments (more than one million visits for all types of complaints performed via telephone, video, or office visits), short-term hospital and ED utilization did not differ between patients who used telemedicine and patients who scheduled in-person visits. This preliminarily suggests that when patients are free to choose their own mode of care within a clinical context that has consistent physicians and ready follow-up care, telemedicine may be a reasonable initial alternative to in-person care and may not lead to increased emergency care. Further research in the same setting as the Reed study showed that e-visits for patients who met specific, low-risk criteria for one of five different complaints (eg, URI, emergency contraception, conjunctivitis, pharyngitis, and urinary tract infections) had overall low rates of in-office follow-up (about 13.5% of the entire cohort), and less than 1% used emergency services.[45] The e-visits took about two to three minutes of clinician time, suggesting this could be a very cost-effective and efficient intervention for common low-acuity complaints.

Even asynchronous patient-physician communication could be a timely way to reduce the need for more intensive care. Patient access to physician-patient messaging through a secure portal may not decrease face-to-face visits overall,[46,47] but for those with multiple chronic conditions (in this study defined as diabetes plus another chronic condition, such as asthma, coronary artery disease, congestive heart failure, or hypertension), it can decrease ED and hospital utilization.[47] This may be particularly significant during times when hospital care is severely overburdened, such as flu seasons, pandemics, or natural disasters. However, increased care burden may fall on outpatient clinicians handling the message volume and could contribute to fatigue or burnout over time if not addressed.

A key health outcome for telemedicine visits that has not been well studied is the diagnostic accuracy of telemedicine evaluation compared with standard care, and the association of delayed diagnosis and adverse health outcomes with each modality. Delayed diagnosis is a frequent allegation in malpractice claims, and to date, the medical-legal footprint of telemedicine has been very small.[48] The medical-legal implications of telemedicine are limited at the time of this publication and will certainly be an area of future research.

SUMMARY AND FUTURE DIRECTIONS

As we prepare to enter a future with widespread telemedicine, we should consider what will be gained and what may be lost. The benefits of telemedicine after its pandemic renaissance are apparent now more than ever: convenient and timely access to care that overcomes geographic barriers, reduced burden on medical infrastructure (e.g., traffic, facilities' wear, perhaps reduced staff needs), and minimal exposure to infectious diseases for all participants. However, concerns still exist that something may be lost if telemedicine becomes standard practice for all. Many telehealth investigators and enthusiasts assert that telemedicine should play a role as an adjunct rather than a replacement for in-person care.[48] This is certainly the most likely scenario, because pandemic restrictions have lessened at the time of authorship of this article, and it remains unclear whether payment parity and other legislation supporting telemedicine care will remain in effect long term. It seems clear thattelemedicine is likely to remain pervasive in some fashion, and this author's review of telemedicine both prepandemic and during the pandemic shows that it is widely agreeable to those who use it and it can stand alongside standard care for a variety of acute and chronic medical conditions, with the opportunity for more research ready to be explored in the future.

Going forward, many questions remain ripe for study on what makes for an effective telemedicine encounter. The relative importance of a physical examination in general and for what types of concerns will need to be considered, as well as to what extent patient-provided vital signs and physician-directed virtual examinations can fill this need. Beyond the physical examination, it is not clear whether patient-clinician relationships, rapport, and trust will suffer through the loss of nonverbal communication and therapeutic touch. Technology challenges from all directions, including poor reception, blurry screen resolution, or choppy Internet connections, may impair the telemedicine rapport. Questions on the impact of telemedicine to specific aspects of the physician-patient relationship deserve further study, as patient adherence and outcomes are known to be heavily influenced by physician communication techniques.[49–52] Perhaps tried-and-true patient communication techniques that have been successfully used in traditional practice to improve patient care[53] can translate relatively easily into telemedicine care and show similar benefits.

It will be to everyone's benefit to understand how to participate in telemedicine care most effectively,as telemedicine is projected to remain more widely available to Americans moving forward. It is time for all of us to become adept at the twenty-first-century house call.

CLINICS CARE POINTS

- Telemedicine use between physicians and patients of all types has greatly expanded with the arrival of the COVID-19 pandemic. It is predicted to remain more prevalent in future US health care.

- Patients who are older, are non-white, live in a rural area, or are from a lower socioeconomic group continue to use telemedicine at lower rates. Some of this inequity is due to inconsistent technology access, but more research is needed in this area.

- Telemedicine is generally well liked by patients who use it, both before and during the pandemic.

- Research supports a role for telemedicine in both acute care and chronic disease management and suggests that it is noninferior to in-person care for health outcomes in certain conditions, such as uncomplicated upper respiratory tract infection, urinary tract infection, low-back pain, initial dermatologic concerns (with the help of high-definition photography), and chronic disease management (with the strongest evidence to date being for diabetes care). Telemedicine may also decrease, or at least not add to, short-term hospital and emergency department utilization.

- Systems-level interventions are needed to solidify telemedicine as a fixture in American health care and ensure more equitable access to it, including more universal service and payment parity, expanded broadband and digital technology access to patients and practices, and the allowance of audio-only telemedicine visits as an acceptable alternative to video.

- Clinicians have cited lack of training as a barrier to practicing telemedicine, and more robust training is needed at the undergraduate and graduate medical education levels. The Association of American Medical Colleges has released telehealth competencies to guide these efforts, and the Society of Teachers of Family Medicine has spearheaded the development of a national telemedicine curriculum.

- Areas of future study should include the development of telemedicine best practices for common acute and chronic conditions and examination of how they affect patient-oriented health outcomes, assessment of physician communication techniques that are suited to remote and audio-only care, study of the economic impact of providing telemedicine care either as adjunct to or in place of in-person care, and the provision of telemedicine access to less represented groups.

DISCLOSURE

None.

REFERENCES

1. Sood S, Mbarika V, Jugoo S, et al. What Is Telemedicine? A Collection of 104 Peer-Reviewed Perspectives and Theoretical Underpinnings. Telemed J E Health 2007;13(5):573–90.
2. Weigel G, Ramaswamy A, May 11 MFP. Opportunities and Barriers for Telemedicine in the U.S. During the COVID-19 Emergency and Beyond. KFF. Published May 11, 2020. 2020. Available at: https://www.kff.org/womens-health-policy/issue-brief/opportunities-and-barriers-for-telemedicine-in-the-u-s-during-the-covid-19-emergency-and-beyond/. Accessed December 21, 2021.
3. Telehealth Is Here to Stay—In the United States and in Germany. AICGS. Available at: https://www.aicgs.org/2020/06/telehealth-is-here-to-stay-in-the-united-states-and-in-germany/. Accessed December 7, 2021.
4. Hyder MA, Razzak J. Telemedicine in the United States: An Introduction for Students and Residents. J Med Internet Res 2020;22(11):e20839.
5. Kane CK, Gillis K. The Use Of Telemedicine By Physicians: Still The Exception Rather Than The Rule. Health Aff (Millwood) 2018;37(12):1923–30.
6. Huilgol YS, Miron-Shatz T, Joshi AU, et al. Hospital Telehealth Adoption Increased in 2014 and 2015 and Was Influenced by Population, Hospital, and Policy Characteristics. Telemed J E Health 2020;26(4):455–61.
7. Ranganathan C, Balaji S. Key Factors Affecting the Adoption of Telemedicine by Ambulatory Clinics: Insights from a Statewide Survey. Telemed J E Health 2020;26(2):218–25.

8. Polinski JM, Barker T, Gagliano N, et al. Patients' Satisfaction with and Preference for Telehealth Visits. J Gen Intern Med 2016;31(3):269–75.

9. Kruse CS, Krowski N, Rodriguez B, et al. Telehealth and patient satisfaction: a systematic review and narrative analysis. BMJ Open 2017;7(8):e016242.

10. Pflugeisen BM, Mou J. Patient Satisfaction with Virtual Obstetric Care. Matern Child Health J 2017;21(7):1544–51.

11. Karen Donelan S, Esteban A, Barreto MA, et al. Patient and Clinician Experiences With Telehealth for Patient Follow-up Care. Published online January 14, 2019. Available at: https://www.ajmc.com/view/patient-and-clinician-experiences-with-telehealth-for-patient-followup-care. Accessed December 9, 2021.

12. Orlando JF, Beard M, Kumar S. Systematic review of patient and caregivers' satisfaction with telehealth videoconferencing as a mode of service delivery in managing patients' health. PLoS One 2019;14(8):e0221848.

13. Hsu H, Greenwald PW, Clark S, et al. Telemedicine Evaluations for Low-Acuity Patients Presenting to the Emergency Department: Implications for Safety and Patient Satisfaction. Telemed J E Health 2020;26(8):1010–5.

14. Haluza D, Naszay M, Stockinger A, et al. Prevailing Opinions on Connected Health in Austria: Results from an Online Survey. Int J Environ Res Public Health 2016;13(8):813.

15. Klink K, Coffman M, Moore M, et al. Family Physician and Telehealth: Findings from a National Survey. Robert Graham Center; 2015. Available at: https://www.graham-center.org/content/dam/rgc/documents/publications-reports/reports/RGC%202015%20Telehealth%20Report.pdf. Accessed February 4, 2022.

16. Weiner JP, Bandeian S, Hatef E, et al. In-Person and Telehealth Ambulatory Contacts and Costs in a Large US Insured Cohort Before and During the COVID-19 Pandemic. JAMA Netw Open 2021;4(3):e212618.

17. Doximity. 2020 State of Telemedicine Report: Examining Patient Perspectives and Physician Adoption of Telemedicine Since the COVID-19 Pandemic. Published online September 2020. Available at: https://c8y.doxcdn.com/image/upload/Press%20Blog/Research%20Reports/2020-state-telemedicine-report.pdf. Accessed December 10, 2021.

18. Patel SY, Mehrotra A, Huskamp HA, et al. Variation In Telemedicine Use And Outpatient Care During The COVID-19 Pandemic In The United States. Health Aff (Millwood) 2021;40(2):349–58.

19. COVID-19 financial impact on physician practices | American Medical Association. Available at: https://www.ama-assn.org/practice-management/sustainability/covid-19-financial-impact-physician-practices. Accessed February 2, 2022.

20. FAIRHealth Monthly Telehealth Regional Tracker. fairhealth.org. Available at: http://www.fairhealth.org/states-by-the-numbers/telehealth. Accessed December 7, 2021.

21. Drake C, Lian T, Cameron B, et al. Understanding Telemedicine's "New Normal": Variations in Telemedicine Use by Specialty Line and Patient Demographics. Telemed J E Health 2021. https://doi.org/10.1089/tmj.2021.0041. tmj.2021.0041.

22. SHADAC analysis of the American Community Survey (ACS) Public Use Microdata Sample (PUMS) files. State Health Compare, SHADAC, University of Minnesota. Available at: statehealthcompare.shadac.org. Accessed December 21, 2021.

23. Eberly LA, Kallan MJ, Julien HM, et al. Patient Characteristics Associated With Telemedicine Access for Primary and Specialty Ambulatory Care During the COVID-19 Pandemic. JAMA Netw Open 2020;3(12):e2031640.

24. Gilson SF, Umscheid CA, Laiteerapong N, et al. Growth of Ambulatory Virtual Visits and Differential Use by Patient Sociodemographics at One Urban Academic Medical Center During the COVID-19 Pandemic: Retrospective Analysis. JMIR Med Inform 2020;8(12):e24544.

25. Hsiao V, Chandereng T, Lankton RL, et al. Disparities in Telemedicine Access: A Cross-Sectional Study of a Newly Established Infrastructure during the COVID-19 Pandemic. Appl Clin Inform 2021;12(3):445–58.

26. Rodriguez JA, Saadi A, Schwamm LH, et al. Disparities In Telehealth Use Among California Patients With Limited English Proficiency: Study examines disparities in telehealth use among California patients with limited English proficiency. Health Aff (Millwood) 2021;40(3):487–95.

27. Research Shows Patients and Clinicians Rated Telemedicine Care Positively During COVID-19 Pandemic - Penn Medicine. Available at: https://www.pennmedicine.org/news/news-releases/2020/june/patients-and-clinicians-rated-telemedicine-care-positively-during-covid. Accessed December 14, 2021.

28. Holtz BE. Patients Perceptions of Telemedicine Visits Before and After the Coronavirus Disease 2019 Pandemic. Telemed J E Health 2021;27(1):107–12.

29. Kyle MA, Blendon RJ, Findling MG, et al. Telehealth use and Satisfaction among U.S. Households: Results of a National Survey. J Patient Exp 2021;8. 23743735211052736.

30. Bashshur RL, Howell JD, Krupinski EA, et al. The Empirical Foundations of Telemedicine Interventions in Primary Care. Telemed J E Health 2016;22(5):342–75.

31. Chaudhry R, Stroebel R, McLeod T, et al. Nurse-based telephone protocol versus usual care for management of URI and acute sinusitis: a controlled trial. Manag Care Interf 2006;19(8):26–31.

32. Stroebel R, McLeod T, Kitsteiner J, et al. Clinical outcomes of patients with upper respiratory tract infections and acute sinusitis managed with a Web-based protocol in primary care practice. Manag Care Interf 2007;20(6):17–22.

33. Uscher-Pines L, Mulcahy A, Cowling D, et al. Access and Quality of Care in Direct-to-Consumer Telemedicine. Telemed J E Health 2016;22(4):282–7.

34. Foster CB, Martinez KA, Sabella C, et al. Patient Satisfaction and Antibiotic Prescribing for Respiratory Infections by Telemedicine. Pediatrics 2019;144(3): e20190844.

35. Ray KN, Shi Z, Gidengil CA, et al. Antibiotic Prescribing During Pediatric Direct-to-Consumer Telemedicine Visits. Pediatrics 2019;143(5):e20182491.

36. Reed M, Huang J, Graetz I, et al. Treatment and Follow-up Care Associated With Patient-Scheduled Primary Care Telemedicine and In-Person Visits in a Large Integrated Health System. JAMA Netw Open 2021;4(11):e2132793.

37. Trettel A, Eissing L, Augustin M. Telemedicine in dermatology: findings and experiences worldwide - a systematic literature review. J Eur Acad Dermatol Venereol 2018;32(2):215–24.

38. Niznik JD, He H, Kane-Gill SL. Impact of clinical pharmacist services delivered via telemedicine in the outpatient or ambulatory care setting: A systematic review. Res Soc Adm Pharm 2018;14(8):707–17.

39. Thomas AM, Baker JW, Hoffmann TJ, et al. Clinical pharmacy specialists providing consistent comprehensive medication management with increased efficiency through telemedicine during the COVID19 pandemic. J Am Coll Clin Pharm 2021;4(8):934–8.

40. Appel LJ, Clark JM, Yeh HC, et al. Comparative Effectiveness of Weight-Loss Interventions in Clinical Practice. N Engl J Med 2011;365(21):1959–68.

41. Kroenke K, Krebs EE, Wu J, et al. Telecare Collaborative Management of Chronic Pain in Primary Care: A Randomized Clinical Trial. JAMA 2014;312(3):240–8.
42. Portnoy JM, Waller M, Lurgio SD, et al. Telemedicine is as effective as in-person visits for patients with asthma. Ann Allergy Asthma Immunol 2016;117(3):241–5.
43. Davies B, Kenia P, Nagakumar P, et al. Paediatric and adolescent asthma: A narrative review of telemedicine and emerging technologies for the post-COVID-19 era. Clin Exp Allergy 2021;51(3):393–401.
44. Timpel P, Oswald S, Schwarz PEH, et al. Mapping the evidence on the effectiveness of telemedicine interventions in diabetes, dyslipidemia, and hypertension: an umbrella review of systematic reviews and meta-analyses. J Med Internet Res 2020;22(3):e16791.
45. Bhargava R, Gayre G, Huang J, et al. Patient e-Visit Use and Outcomes for Common Symptoms in an Integrated Health Care Delivery System. JAMA Netw Open 2021;4(3):e212174.
46. North F, Crane SJ, Chaudhry R, et al. Impact of Patient Portal Secure Messages and Electronic Visits on Adult Primary Care Office Visits. Telemed J E Health 2014;20(3):192–8.
47. Reed ME, Huang J, Brand RJ, et al. Patients with complex chronic conditions: Health care use and clinical events associated with access to a patient portal. PLoS One 2019;14(6):e0217636.
48. The Doctors Company. Your Patient Is Logging On Now: The Risks and Benefits of Telehealth in the Future of Healthcare. The Doctors Company TDC Group. Available at: https://www.thedoctors.com/articles/your-patient-is-logging-on-now–the-risks-and-benefits-of-telehealth-in-the-future-of-healthcare/. Accessed December 21, 2021.
49. Stewart MA. Effective physician-patient communication and health outcomes: a review. CMAJ Can Med Assoc J 1995;152(9):1423–33.
50. Levinson W, Roter DL, Mullooly JP, et al. Physician-patient communication: The relationship with malpractice claims among primary care physicians and surgeons. JAMA 1997;277(7):553–9.
51. Haskard Zolnierek KB, DiMatteo MR. Physician Communication and Patient Adherence to Treatment: A Meta-analysis. Med Care 2009;47(8):826–34.
52. Strumann C, Steinhaeuser J, Emcke T, et al. Communication training and the prescribing pattern of antibiotic prescription in primary health care. PLoS One 2020;15(5):e0233345.
53. Stein T. A Decade of Experience with a Multiday Residential Communication Skills Intensive: Has the Outcome Been Worth the Investment? Perm J 2007;11(4):30–40.

Asynchronous Telehealth

Jennifer Stephens, DO, MBA[a], Grant M. Greenberg, MD, MA, MHSA[b],*

KEYWORDS

- E-consults • Virtual consultation • Asynchronous telemedicine • E-visits

KEY POINTS

- Asynchronous telehealth, which includes both e-visits and e-consults, refers to the "store-and-forward" technique, in which a patient or clinician collects and reports medical information and then sends it to a health care provider for diagnosis and treatment recommendations.
- The highest utility for e-visits is for lower acuity illness that does not require immediate evaluation and for which diagnosis does not require a physical examination.
- The potential benefits of asynchronous telehealth e-consultation between primary care and subspecialty care providers depend on the nature and framework of the local implementation, the breadth of available subspecialties, and the ability of the primary care physician to follow through on the recommendation provided by the subspecialist.
- Asynchronous virtual care is recognized for providing scale, value, and efficiency. Tracking volume, turnaround time, and quality variables involved in service delivery are critically important in ensuring patient satisfaction, programmatic success, and sustainability.

INTRODUCTION/HISTORY

Although traditional health care is nearly always delivered in a synchronous format, telehealth delivery can be either synchronous or asynchronous. All forms of synchronous medical care, from a patient perspective, involve traveling to a medical facility or logging onto a technological platform, sitting in a waiting room (brick and mortar or virtual), and receiving care from a physician or advanced-practice clinician in an "examination room." This model of care requires coordination of the schedules for both the patient and clinician and ready availability of either technology or a facility that is both equipped and staffed. Many potential constraints to synchronous medical care occur, and consequently, patients sometimes cancel, reschedule, or do not come for care at the recommended interval (**Table 1**).

[a] Lehigh Valley Physician Group, Lehigh Valley Health Network, LVHN-One City Center, 707 Hamilton Street – 7th Floor, PO Box 1806, Allentown, PA 18105-1806, USA; [b] Lehigh Valley Health Network, LVHN-One City Center, 707 Hamilton Street - 8th Floor, PO Box 1806, Allentown, PA 18105-1806, USA
* Corresponding author.
E-mail address: Grant.Greenberg@LVHN.org

Prim Care Clin Office Pract 49 (2022) 531–541
https://doi.org/10.1016/j.pop.2022.05.004
0095-4543/22/© 2022 Elsevier Inc. All rights reserved.
primarycare.theclinics.com

Table 1	
Potential patient constraints limiting access to medical care	
Synchronous Face-to-Face Care Barriers	**Synchronous Virtual Care Barriers**
Geographic proximity to the desired medical care	Technology availability at the exact time of scheduled appointment
Ability to take time off work	Ability to find private location for visit
Access to transportation	Access to technology
Clinician schedule and appointment access that matches needs	
Physical or cognitive limitations	
Challenges in arranging child-care	

Synchronous consultation from a primary care clinician perspective also includes a multitude of challenges in terms of garnering information from requested consultants. These challenges include many of the same constraints from a patient perspective, including geographic proximity of the patient to the selected subspecialty consultant, timely access to that consultant, and actionable communication regarding the subsequent recommended care.

In this article, the authors discuss the use of asynchronous telehealth in the form of e-visits and e-consults. The concept of telehealth has been in existence for close to 100 years.[1] Technology only imagined in the 1920s has become the reality of the 2020s with a dizzying and rapid development linked to the explosion of worldwide technology; this includes the ubiquitous nature of the Internet, hand-held/portable personal data devices (eg, iPhones, iPads, and so forth), electronic medical records (EMRs), and computerized data and analytical systems. The development of technology has actualized the potential to relieve patients and clinicians from the constraints of traditional health care and to use telehealth in both synchronous and asynchronous fashions.

DEFINITIONS/BACKGROUND

Asynchronous telehealth, which includes both e-visits and e-consults, refers to the "store-and-forward" technique, in which a patient or clinician collects and reports medical information and then sends it to a health care provider for diagnosis and treatment recommendations.[2] With the advent of e-mail, and patient access to "portals" through an EMR, informal requests and communications from patients for advice is a common cited "burden" contributing to clinician burnout (**Box 1**). As an example of this is a study that originated from the Palo Alto Medical Foundation group; they surveyed their physicians across primary care and specialty areas and found that receipt of an above-average number of in-basket messages was associated with 40% increase in the risk for burnout.[3]

Box 1
Types of asynchronous communication

- E-visit: billable asynchronous virtual visit between patient and clinician
- E-consult: billable asynchronous virtual consult between clinicians
- E-mail: nonbillable communication message between patient and clinician

Unlike informal e-mail messages, an e-visit consists of a structured set of predefined questions designed to gather enough information to facilitate diagnosis and treatment without the need for a real-time interaction with a patient. In addition, in many systems a patient can upload photographs or even video recordings to facilitate a more robust evaluation and management paradigm. An e-visit typically originates from the patient and is directed to the clinician. Clinicians can, however, convert an e-mail into a billable e-visit if warranted, clinically appropriate, and patient consent is obtained.

An e-consult is typically initiated by a clinician and is directed to another clinician, typically a primary care physician to a subspecialty consultant. In this model of care, a primary care physician can submit an electronic request within the EMR to a subspecialty consultant. The subspecialty consultant, in turn, can access the information available within the medical record and respond with specific advice for evaluation, management, and follow-up directly to the primary care physician. As this asynchronous information exchange occurs within the medical record, it replaces what is known as a "curbside consult" and is a billable service. The patient benefits as they receive the input of a subspecialist without need for travel, and although expectations vary, a response can occur rapidly (**Box 2** on general turnaround time guidelines). Recognizing the potential of this model to enhance access to subspecialists for higher acuity patients, in 2014 the Association of American Medical Colleges initiated a program called Project CORE "Coordinating Optimal Referral Experiences."[4] Project CORE has expanded to include more than 40 Academic Medical Systems, and many other institutions now provide a similar model of consultation (**Fig. 1**).

OUTCOMES
E-Visit Outcomes

A systematic review of asynchronous electronic communication in patients with chronic conditions demonstrated improvement in self-management and health outcomes such as the control of diabetes, hypertension, and asthma. De Jong and colleagues[5] conducted a systemic review of 15 studies that evaluated asynchronous communication between patients and providers and found an overall improvement in HbA1C levels, blood pressure control, forced expiratory volume in the first second of expiration, and asthma control. Given the difference in methodology across the included studies, the magnitude of improvement was difficult to consistently quantify but the use of electronic communication was the unifying feature.

Despite the convenience and opportunity to receive care without a visit, one study found that contrary to expectation, e-visit utilization generated a higher number of office visits and decreased access for new patients.[6] This study evaluated 140,000 patients across 90 providers over a 5-year period and noted that e-visits triggered an

---

Box 2
General turnaround time guidelines

- In all scenarios, the faster the response is ideal.
- Acute urgent care e-visit: ideal response within 1 to 2 hours, no longer than 6 hours
- Primary care e-visit: response within 24 hours, no longer than 48 hours
- Email to established clinician: response within 24 hours, no longer than 48 hours
- E-consult: response within 48 hours, no longer than 72 hours

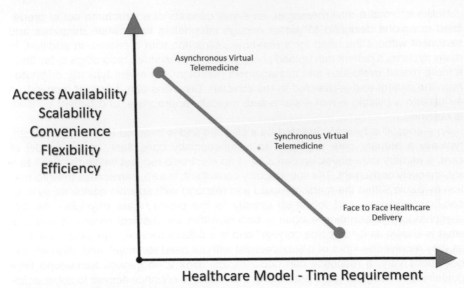

Fig. 1. Theoretic health care delivery construct for access versus time. (*Courtesy of* Jen Stephens, DO, MBA, FACP, Allentown, PA.)

incremental 6% to 7% volume of office visits and telephone encounters. Because e-visits go directly to the physician, the lack of a "gatekeeper" resulted in a higher number of subsequent visits and consequently a reduction of available appointments for new patients. Further and ongoing evaluation may be needed to confirm or inform factors that can both provide convenience without increasing task burden or decreasing overall access. Before the Sars-CoV-2 pandemic, e-visit adaptation was growing in the United States, with up to 15.9% of physicians using this technology in 2015.[7] Not surprisingly, the strongest predictor of adoption of e-visits was a fully implemented EMR (odds ratio 2.66), whereas other factors included a capitated payment model.

Evidence suggests that the clinical care provided in an e-visit can offer equivalent clinical outcome as that provided by synchronous care. Nguyen and colleagues[8] conducted a systemic review of published studies on e-visit outcomes spanning the past 20 years. Included studies reported on clinical outcomes, health care quality, access, utilization, or costs and were not specific to any specialty or condition. Although most of the included studies were small, outcomes such as glucose control and anticoagulation management were superior in e-visits, whereas there was lower utilization of diagnostic procedures for evaluation of urinary tract infection and sinusitis. However, not all was positive, as there was also a lower rate of preventive screening and a higher utilization of antibiotics for sinusitis. The highest utility for e-visits seems to be for lower acuity illness that does not require immediate evaluation and for which diagnosis does not require a physical examination.[9] Lastly, it is not clear that all patients can readily access asynchronous telehealth. Some patients may lack the resources to access an EMR, whereas others may have cognitive or physical disability[10] or be elderly, with associated limitations in virtual engagement.[11]

Patient experience of care with asynchronous telehealth visits has not been well reported. The continued use and expansion of commercial entities as well as health systems offering this as an option speaks to patient demand. However, further analysis of patient outcomes and experience is still under development. Hickson and colleagues[12] note that analyses of e-visits are typically lacking analysis of patient satisfaction and there is need for future evaluation of this area, which is insufficiently studied to date.

E-Consult Outcomes

One of the primary outcomes desired from asynchronous telehealth consultations when originated was to improve access and decrease consultation delays. Although anecdotal and personal experience confirm that outcome, research to date through randomized controlled trial and meta-analytic evidence is insufficient to validate this concept.[13] Despite this, there is still strong support for benefit to timely access to specialty care and engagement and usage by primary care physicians. Vimalananda and colleagues[14] conducted a meta-analysis on studies published between 1990 and 2014 related to e-consults. They found that primary care physicians were highly satisfied with the convenience, value, and access to specialties through e-consults. However, although specialists found e-consults beneficial to reduce inappropriate clinic visits and improve efficiency when initial testing was completed before a visit, there was some concern about potential liability providing advice on a patient who had never been seen in person. Given that, if the new process is viewed as beneficial with significant intrinsic value to the clinician and patient, the uptake will likely be higher.

In the case of asynchronous telehealth consultation, factors that predict successful implementation include strong primary care–subspecialist relationships,[15] reliable and compatible technology, effective training, and effective dissemination of information.[16] Another key factor that can predict successful application is a consistent response time by the subspecialist to the primary care physician placing the asynchronous telehealth consultation.[17] The potential benefits of asynchronous telehealth e-consultation likely depend on the nature of the local implementation, the breadth of available subspecialties, and the ability of the primary care physician to follow through on the recommendation supplied by the specialist. A summary of potential benefits to this method of consultation is summarized in **Box 3**.

OPERATIONAL CONSIDERATIONS

The implementation of virtual asynchronous telehealth services requires consideration of multiple operational factors for successful deployment and sustainability. These factors include workforce, standard guidelines, process and workflow, data analytics, reimbursement, and technology. Each element is worthy of attention and if not optimized, can cause potential disruption in experience, safety, and outcomes.

Structured questions are a necessary part of a successful e-visit. Because the e-visit, by definition, does not provide an opportunity for an interactive discourse between a physician and patient, obtaining the essential elements in the form of directed data input from a patient is mandatory. EMRs that offer e-visits within the programming may have templates to facilitate e-visits developed by clinician input. The type of question, content, and level of detail will vary across settings. In addition, questions should be used to minimize the risk of topics not appropriate for e-visit (ie, "Do you have chest pain? If so, please call 911."). The most common topics seen by e-visit tend to be low-acuity conditions such as urinary tract infection and sinusitis.[9] It may be possible, based on local licensure rules, to have staff or nursing protocols developed for common, simple diagnoses managed on an e-visit. However, even if allowed, a licensed physician is still required to provide oversight for medical decision-making. In addition, topics such as tobacco cessation, hypertension management, and follow-up for stable, chronic conditions are also potentially appropriate for asynchronous telehealth.

> **Box 3**
> **Benefits of asynchronous telehealth consultation**
>
> - Decreased clinic wait times for those still seeking in-person care[18]
> - Reduction in traditional referrals (hence enhancing access)[19]
> - Decreased travel burden and travel costs for patients[20]
> - Development of knowledge and professional development of the primary care physician in the specialty topic[21]
> - Reduced wait times for specialty consultation coupled with increased referral completion rates[22]
> - Improved access to specialty care for underserved populations[23]
> - Reduced specialty utilization[25,26]
> - Reduced cost of care[24]

Obtaining an effective e-consult through asynchronous telehealth requires clarity of the question being asked, availability of the relevant information in the medical record, and ability for the primary care physician to follow through on the recommendations in a timely manner.[25] Guidance to the primary care physician from the subspecialist within the e-consult request or order can facilitate higher quality, more effective consultation. Tools that provide guidelines can be robust and potentially incorporated into the EMR.[26]

Workforce

Each organization or practice needs to define the clinician workforce providing the asynchronous care. Depending on the visit type and clinician scenario prompting the telehealth encounter, the workforce may be decentralized and specific, or may be more centralized and overseen at a higher level within an organization. An e-visit sent to a primary care clinician may be managed directly by that individual, whereas some practice locations or organizations may centralize management of all e-visits (for urgent care e-visits for example) to ensure timely response or to leverage a team-based and standardized approach to care. This structure depends on each individual system's approach to virtual offerings, clinician scheduling, and task management.

Removing the element of synchronized, timed requirements allows a workforce to be pooled with multiple assigned individuals for coverage. This model works well in acute e-visit settings and in scenarios where large encounter volumes are anticipated with little required linkage to chronic condition management. The COVID-19 pandemic provided a strong example of this situation. When the pandemic began, there was a need for immediate deployment of telehealth COVID-19 screening visits to provide virtual availability to the community. This demand required rapid workforce deployment to navigate an overnight incremental push for service delivery. In some organizations, the e-visit model allowed for immediate expansion of service delivery without a concomitant brick and mortar or extensive rescheduling requirement. The asynchronous nature of the e-visit telehealth model allowed a large group of primary care clinicians and advanced-practice clinicians to support this demand remotely while still completing their traditional daily office duties. The management and oversight of this clinical service offering was performed centrally, leveraging a large and rapidly deployed remote workforce to meet the needs of a large community demand through e-visit asynchronous care.

As the pandemic example demonstrated, if the established time standards for the virtual telehealth response are met, the clinician staffing model can be flexible and allow for clinician response to visits or consults at any hour of day or night. This flexibility can be a recruitment tool for those clinicians seeking alternative schedules and remote work opportunities.

Either way, it is important for an organization to assign responsibility and expectations around response times and clinician coverage to avoid any gaps in care and ensure patient safety. If clinical staff are involved in the routing of virtual encounters, clear expectations around their communication with patients and workflow with covering clinicians must be defined.

Standard Guidelines

With all the benefits that asynchronous care provides in convenience and scalability, the lack of real-time dialogue allowing clarification of clinical content can create risk. A standard guideline document clearly outlining expectations around patient's expected response times and clinical management principles can mitigate this risk. These management principles can be individualized to each clinical organization and can range from expectations around analgesic prescribing for pain complaints (ie, not allowing opioids to be prescribed unless a face-to-face visit occurs) to antibiotic prescribing for sinus symptoms (ie, supporting prescribing only when certain clinical parameters are met). Standardized templates can then be developed, driven from virtual clinical encounter offerings (eg, acute complaints for urgent care e-visit offerings), to assist patient symptom evaluation and limit downstream clarifications that may be required. See Appendix for an example template questionnaire used during COVID-19 pandemic for e-visit guidance.

Clear communication to patients about expected response time and what situations are not appropriate for asynchronous encounters is just as important as a standard document for clinicians. Efforts should be taken to transparently communicate that guidance to patients before the encounter is begun to avoid delays in care and risk to patients due to inappropriate triage direction. An example of this would be a patient submitting an e-visit online with a potential 24-hour turnaround time for a complaint of chest pain or acute stroke symptoms. Organizations should consider having staff triage all asynchronous messages to ensure appropriateness and timely management. That added workflow element promotes enhanced patient safety, given the time delay inherent in this model of care.

Included in standard guidelines is the expectation around a core set of patient education and communication materials. Ensuring a consistent clinical model of care is delivered via the asynchronous telehealth model will provide enhanced patient safety and a platform on which to reliably evaluate clinical outcomes.

Technology

Health care organizations interested in providing virtual asynchronous telehealth services must have an EMR system with requisite functionality or a technology partner with those capabilities. At a minimum, the required platform must be HIPAA secure and perform as a 2-way communication portal. Billing capabilities should be included, with reimbursement and coding tools available. Compliance and legal guidance should direct the start-up of these programs, given the ever-changing landscape of telehealth and payer contract coverage models.

Although apparent, a key prerequisite to patient completion of an asynchronous virtual telehealth encounter is the availability of a phone or device that can access the

Internet. Leveraging these technologies expands access to many more patients across our communities than modalities that require a computer or laptop-type device.

Process/Workflow

Defining response timelines for an organization should be tied to the nature of the clinical service offering, workforce available, and day/time of the week. An acute urgent care type e-visit should have a more rapid turnaround time compared with a chronic condition follow-up e-visit that is sent to a primary care clinician. In all scenarios, clear expectations regarding response times should be conveyed to patients as they submit their encounter requests.

Data/Analytics

Monitoring performance in any initiative requires tracking of data and analysis of impact. In developing programs around asynchronous virtual telehealth, metrics should be framed around operational elements, reimbursement performance, and any other area that an organization feels reflects success. It is recommended that clinical leadership is involved in informatics and data analytics to guide many of these elements.

Reimbursement

The current landscape for virtual care reimbursement is ever-evolving. Many asynchronous telehealth visits are billed based on time factors required for completion of the encounter. Coverage is payer dependent and variable depending on geography. The Medicare Physician Fee Schedule final rule describes e-visits as non–face-to-face "patient initiated digital communications that require a clinical decision that otherwise typically would have been provided in the office." CMS[27] has established specific billing requirements: the patient must be established with the office and initiate contact through a patient portal; they must consent to the e-visit; time spent reviewing, assessing, and responding over the next 7 days determines the level of service with appropriate supportive documentation. **Table 2** delineates specific current procedural terminology (CPT) codes and work relative value unites (wRVU) values for e-visits.

RISKS

Although asynchronous telehealth has clear advantages and benefits, there are also significant drawbacks. Among them, as described by Kaplan[28] include some depersonalization of the patient care experience. There is a risk for communication gaps

Table 2
CPT codes and wRVU values

CPT Code	Description	wRVU Value (Nonfacility)
99421	Online digital evaluation and management service for an established patient, for up to 7 d, cumulative time during the 7 d; 5–10 min	0.43
99422	Online digital evaluation and management service for an established patient, for up to 7 d, cumulative time during the 7 d; 11–200 min	0.86
99423	Online digital evaluation and management service for an established patient, for up to 7 d, cumulative time during the 7 d; 21 or more minutes	1.39

Data from Centers for Medicare & Medicaid Services. Physician Fee Schedule. December 1, 2021. Accessed December 15, 2021. https://www.cms.gov/Medicare/Medicare-Fee-for-Service-Payment/PhysicianFeeSched.

due to technology access, function, or patient disability or cognitive function. The lack of a physical examination may result in degradation of the integrity of information obtained to guide medical decisions. Concerns about privacy include cybersecurity and risk for loss of patient confidentiality without control of the patient's visit environment. Liability/malpractice risk is always a concern for any medical care, and asynchronous care is no exception. Mitigating liability through structured visits and patient consent in advance, acknowledging the limits of the scope, are reasonable measures to institute. Lastly, the economic sustainability of asynchronous telehealth depends, in part, on reimbursement approval by payors, CMS, and on the patient side acceptance that some topics will require in-person follow-up.

SUMMARY

Asynchronous telehealth in the form of e-visits and e-consults is an effective tool that provides benefit to both patients and physicians. Improved efficiency, access, and convenience are balanced by loss of interactive information gathering and human contact. When technology is available to support asynchronous telehealth, there are benefits to both the physicians and the patients. These benefits are summarized in the following section.

CLINICS CARE POINTS

- Asynchronous telehealth, which includes both e-visits and e-consults, refers to the "store-and-forward" technique, in which a patient or clinician collects and reports medical information and then sends it to a health care provider for diagnosis and treatment recommendations.

- E-visit: billable asynchronous virtual visit between patient and clinician.

- E-consult: billable asynchronous virtual consult between clinician and clinician.

- E-mail: nonbillable communication message between patient and clinician.

- The highest utility for e-visits seems to be for lower acuity illness that does not require immediate evaluation and for which diagnosis does not require a physical examination.

- The potential benefits of asynchronous telehealth e-consultation likely depend on the nature of the local implementation, the breadth of available specialties, and the ability of the primary care physician to follow through on the recommendation supplied by the specialist.

- Key operational factors include workforce, standard guidelines, process/workflow, data analytics, reimbursement, and technology.

- Clinician staffing models for asynchronous telehealth encounters can often be flexible, acting as a recruitment tool for those clinicians seeking alternative schedules or remote work opportunities.

- Development of a Standard Guideline document outlining explicit management principles can mitigate the inherent risk created from an asynchronous model (secondary to the lack of real-time dialogue allowing clarification of clinical history content).

- At minimum, the required platform must be HIPAA secure and perform as a 2-way communication portal. Asynchronous telehealth can be limited by lack of access to technology and difficulty with navigating technology due to vulnerability, disability, or cognitive functioning.

- Limitations include the potential for communication gaps and language barriers due to the loss of synchronous human interaction. In addition, asynchronous telehealth limits the ability to clarify in real time the information integrity to ensure the most appropriate medical decision-making. This may potentially increase liability and malpractice risk depending on the clinical situation.

- Asynchronous virtual care is recognized for providing scale, value, and efficiency. Tracking volumes, turnaround time, and quality variables involved in service delivery are critically important in ensuring patient satisfaction, programmatic success, and sustainability.

DISCLOSURE

Neither author has any disclosures.

SUPPLEMENTARY DATA

Supplementary data related to this article can be found online at https://doi.org/10.1016/j.pop.2022.05.004.

REFERENCES

1. Smithsonian Magazine, "Telemedicine Predicted in 1925". 2012. Available at: https://www.smithsonianmag.com/history/telemedicine-predicted-in-1925-124140942/. Accessed October 4, 2021.
2.. Mechanic OJ, Persaud Y, Kimball AB. Telehealth systems. In: StatPearls [internet]. Treasure Island (FL): StatPearls Publishing; 2021. p. 1–5. Available at: https://www.ncbi.nlm.nih.gov/books/NBK459384/.
3. Ming TS, Dillon EC, Yan Yang, et al. Physicians' Well-Being Linked To In-Basket Messages Generated By Algorithms In Electronic Health Records. Frosch Health Aff 2019;38(7):1073–8.
4. Available at: https://www.aamc.org/what-we-do/mission-areas/health-care/project-core. Accessed October 4, 2021.
5. de Jong CC, Ros WJ, Schrijvers G. The effects on health behavior and health outcomes of internet-based asynchronous communication between health providers and patients with a chronic condition: A systematic review. J Med Internet Res 2014;16(1):1. https://doi.org/10.2196/jmir.3000. Available at: http://ezproxy.lib.usf.edu/login?url=https://www.proquest.com/scholarly-journals/effects-on-health-behavior-outcomes-internet/docview/1499152704/se-2.
6. Bavafa H, Hitt LM, Terwiesch C. The Impact of E-Visits on Visit Frequencies and Patient Health: Evidence from Primary Care. Manage Sci 2018;64(12):5461–80.
7. Hong YR, Turner K, Yadav S, et al. Trends in e-visit adoption among U.S. office-based physicians: Evidence from the 2011-2015 NAMCS. Int J Med Inf 2019;129:260–6.
8. Nguyen OT, Alishahi Tabriz A, Huo J, et al. Impact of Asynchronous Electronic Communication-Based Visits on Clinical Outcomes and Health Care Delivery: Systematic Review. J Med Internet Res 2021;23(5):e27531.
9. Hertzog R, Johnson J, Smith J, et al. Diagnostic Accuracy in Primary Care E-Visits: Evaluation of a Large Integrated Health Care Delivery System's Experience. Mayo Clin Proc 2019;94(6):976–84.
10. Annaswamy TM, Verduzco-Gutierrez M, Frieden L. Telemedicine barriers and challenges for persons with disabilities: COVID-19 and beyond. Disabil Health J 2020;13(4):100973.
11. Lam K, Lu AD, Shi Y, et al. Assessing Telemedicine Unreadiness Among Older Adults in the United States During the COVID-19 Pandemic. JAMA Intern Med 2020;180(10):1389–91.

12. Hickson R, Talbert J, Thornbury WC, et al. Online medical care: the current state of "eVisits" in acute primary care delivery. Telemed J E Health 2015;21(2):90–6.
13. Wilson AD, Childs S, Gonçalves-Bradley DC, et al. Interventions to increase or decrease the length of primary care physicians' consultation. Cochrane Database Syst Rev 2016;8:CD003540. Accessed November 02 2021.
14. Vimalananda VG, Gupte G, Seraj SM, et al. Electronic consultations (e-consults) to improve access to specialty care: a systematic review and narrative synthesis. J Telemed Telecare 2015;21(6):323–30.
15. Knox M, Murphy EJ, Leslie T, et al. e-Consult implementation success: lessons from 5 county-based delivery systems. Am J Manag Care 2020;26(1):e21–7.
16. Haverhals LM, Sayre G, Helfrich CD, et al. E-consult implementation: lessons learned using consolidated framework for implementation research. Am J Manag Care 2015;21(12):e640–7.
17. Parikh PJ, Mowrey C, Gallimore J, et al. Evaluating e-consultation implementations based on use and time-line across various specialties. Int J Med Inf 2017;108:42–8.
18. Patel V, Stewart D, Horstman MJ. E-consults: an effective way to decrease clinic wait times in rheumatology. BMC Rheumatol 2020;4:54.
19. Wasfy JH, Rao SK, Kalwani N, et al. Longer-term impact of cardiology e-consults. Am Heart J 2016;173:86–93.
20. Kirsh S, Carey E, Aron DC, et al. Impact of a national specialty e-consultation implementation project on access. Am J Manag Care 2015;21(12):e648–54.
21. ran C, Liddy C, Pinto N, et al. Impact of Question Content on e-Consultation Outcomes. Telemed J E Health 2016;22(3):216–22.
22. Schettini P, Shah KP, O'Leary CP, et al. Keeping care connected: e-Consultation program improves access to nephrology care. J Telemed Telecare 2019;25(3): 142–50.
23. Olayiwola JN, Anderson D, Jepeal N, et al. Electronic Consultations to Improve the Primary Care-Specialty Care Interface for Cardiology in the Medically Underserved: A Cluster-Randomized Controlled Trial. Ann Fam Med 2016;14(2): 133–40.
24. Newman ED, Simonelli PF, Vezendy SM, et al. Impact of primary and specialty care integration via asynchronous communication. Am J Manag Care 2019; 25(1):26–31. Available at: http://ezproxy.lib.usf.edu/login?url=https://www.proquest.com/scholarly-journals/impact-primary-specialty-care-integration-via/docview/2179414959/se-2?accountid=1474.
25. Goldman L, Lee T, Rudd P. Ten Commandments for Effective Consultations. Arch Intern Med 1983;143(9):1753–5.
26. University of Michigan Consultation Request Guidelines. PolicyStat. Available at: https://michmed-public.policystat.com/policy_search/?q=crg/.   Accessed December 15 2021.
27. Centers for Medicare & Medicaid Services. Physician Fee Schedule. 2021. Available at: https://www.cms.gov/Medicare/Medicare-Fee-for-Service-Payment/PhysicianFeeSched. Accessed December 15 2021.
28. Kaplan B. Revisiting health information technology ethical, legal, and social issues and evaluation: telehealth/telemedicine and COVID-19. Int J Med Inf 2020;143:104239.

Applications of Remote Patient Monitoring

Robert Kruklitis, MD, PhD, MBA[a],*, Matthew Miller, DO, MBA[b],
Lorraine Valeriano, BSN, CNRN, CHC[a], Steven Shine, BSE[a], Nadine Opstbaum, MBA[a],
Victoria Chestnut, DNP, MBA, RN[a]

KEYWORDS

- Remote patient monitoring • Home tele-monitoring • Home health monitoring
- Telemedicine • Early detection

KEY POINTS

- Technological enhancements now permit ongoing assessment of a patient's health status within their environment.
- The value proposition for remote patient monitoring is to detect early deterioration, resulting in improved clinical outcomes and decreased health care costs.
- Organizations looking to implement remote patient monitoring will have several operational decisions to make, including the use of nurses and support staff, and how the program workflows will be implemented to support goals.
- Financial billing opportunities to support the program have been made available by Medicare, recognizing the value of remote patient monitoring services.

INTRODUCTION

Remote patient monitoring (RPM) programs use digitally transmitted health-related data to improve patient care. Although there are a wide variety of program designs, they share the fundamental goal of improving health-related outcomes and reducing unnecessary health care costs. The Centers for Medicare and Medicaid Services (CMS) defines RPM as "the collection and analysis of patient physiologic data that are used to develop and manage a treatment plan related to a chronic and/or acute health illness or condition."[1] This article reviews the currently available technology used to acquire these data, describes the fundamental features of program design, understands the financial considerations, and discusses common clinical conditions using RPM.

Although the concept of remotely monitoring patients outside of the hospital dates to the 1990s,[2] interest has recently increased. In part, this is due to technological enhancements that permit the monitoring of a patient's health status from a home setting. CMSs decision to reimburse has also contributed to interest, as RPM is

[a] Lehigh Valley Health Network CARES Center, 2024 Lehigh Street, Allentown, PA 18103, USA;
[b] Cleveland Clinic, 9500 Euclid Avenue, Cleveland, OH 44195, USA
* Corresponding author.
E-mail address: robert.kruklitis@LVHN.org

Prim Care Clin Office Pract 49 (2022) 543–555
https://doi.org/10.1016/j.pop.2022.05.005
0095-4543/22/© 2022 Elsevier Inc. All rights reserved.

primarycare.theclinics.com

now seen as a new source of revenue. Many programs are increasingly interested in analyzing biometrical data obtained from their patients. Analytical analysis of these data, used either alone or in combination with other clinical and claims data, is helping to understand and predict a patient's health trajectory. Many see RPM as a means to provide high-quality care to patients, which will be needed to succeed in value-based arrangements.

The goal of RPM is to use digitally transmitted health-related data to improve patient outcomes. Effective monitoring outside of traditional health care settings permits the early identification of deterioration or change in status. Ideally, programs collect and analyze these data looking for evidence of early decompensation. Early detection creates the opportunity for course correction by addressing pertinent issues and mitigating declining health status. Effective programs identify deterioration early enough to successfully intervene, improve clinical outcomes, and lower care costs.

RPM programs are designed to improve patient care. Compared with conventional care, there are several theoretic benefits of RPM:

- Detect decompensation earlier for improved clinical outcomes
- Meet quality goals, such as decreasing emergency department (ED) utilization
- Facilitate ongoing connection with patients
- Better patient education to improve self-management
- Enhance the provider–patient relationship
- Increase patient engagement and satisfaction
- Enhance revenue through new reimbursement options

Whether RPM can reliably deliver value, and under which clinical scenarios, has yet to be proven. Many RPM studies report utilization metrics, such as hospitalizations and ED visits. Other important metrics include health-related quality of life, disease control, and morbidity and mortality. The number of reports highlighting these metrics and other benefits of RPM continues to grow. Given the extensive variability between programs and the limited number of publications, it is difficult to make definitive conclusions regarding the benefit of RPM. Every program is different in terms of biometrics obtained, frequency of data transmission, and interventions used when abnormalities are identified. Further research needs to be conducted to define the optimal program characteristics and the patient population that will most benefit from this service.

Ultimately, the most successful programs capitalize on coordination between clinical, technology, and operational leadership. Clinical leadership drives the design of the use cases, obtains stakeholder engagement, and develops clinical workflows. Technology leadership vets the technical and security attributes of vendors and medical devices under consideration. In addition, technology ensures that the data gathered from RPM are available within the necessary workflows and presented to the clinicians in a meaningful way. Operational leadership focuses on program design and implementation. Key components include managing human and financial resources, creating standard work, maintaining a device deployment/recovery plan, and outlining key performance indicators that support program goals. The overall goal of this article is to provide a framework to understand the various technical, operational, and clinical considerations involved and to provide a review of the common clinical conditions using RPM.

TECHNOLOGICAL CONSIDERATIONS

Technology plays a critical role in forming and maintaining RPM programs. Ensuring that data are reliable and accurate is paramount to guaranteeing clinician and patient confidence with the program. There are two core functions of the technical team: selecting devices and ensuring accurate data delivery.

To accommodate the increased demand for RPM, a growing number of home monitoring devices have recently entered the marketplace. A major decision in establishing an RPM program is the selection of devices. There are several key factors to consider:

1. *Clinical Accuracy*: An effective RPM program uses data to inform clinical decisions. It is critical that the devices provide reliable, accurate information. Clinically reviewed devices, such as those approved by the Food and Drug Administration (FDA) or those on the US Validated Device Listing, are a good place to start.
2. *Security and Health Insurance Portability and Accountability Act (HIPAA)Compliance*: RPM devices allow patient-specific clinical information to be transmitted and are regulated under HIPAA. It is important to understand the flow of clinical information, including where, when, and how the data are encrypted, to maintain HIPAA compliance.
3. *Ease of Use*: The success of an RPM program relies on a patient's ability and willingness to submit data. It is important to ensure that collection, display, and transmission of the clinical data are straightforward, particularly for older patients.
4. *Cost*: The cost of devices can impact the program. With a new focus on consumer grade medical device products, it is increasingly possible to find quality devices at a lower cost.
5. *Stock and Availability*: Ensuring a reliable, steady supply of devices is a key factor during selection. Even small interruptions in device availability can halt a program. Changing devices requires significant work, including testing, updating training materials, and potentially building new integrations.

Another critical consideration is the level of device integration within an electronic medical record (EMR). There are three distinct types of integration:

1. *No integration or manual integration:* Like traditional glucometers, some devices do not support EMR integration. These devices output biometric readings to a screen or indicator built directly on the device. Patients can track readings on a paper log or by manually entering data into a flow sheet or table. Some portals allow patients to manually track this biometric data online by submitting to the EMR.
2. *Bluetooth integration:* Among the fastest-growing device types support Bluetooth integration. These devices record biometric data and transmit it wirelessly to the patient's smartphone. An app on the patient's phone retrieves the readings and logs them over time. Aggregators, such as Apple Health or Google Fit, further support integration by consolidating data from several apps into a central location. Some EMR systems support integration with aggregators to download data directly into the patient's chart.
3. *Cellular/mobile network integration:* The deepest level of integration comes from cellular or mobile network integration. With this setup, a hub device is paired with the patient's EMR. When readings are taken by an accompanying device near the hub, the hub will use either the patient's home wireless network or a cellular network to file the readings directly into the patient's EMR.

When creating an RPM program, it is critical to understand each of these integration options and then weigh each against the goals and funding of the program. The specific devices required will depend on the clinical conditions being monitored; devices

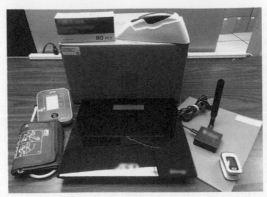

Fig. 1. Sample RPM kit with cellular hub, pulse oximeter, thermometer, scale, and blood pressure monitor. Patient instructions are also included with the kit.

may include blood pressure cuffs, pulse oximeters, scales, glucometers, or thermometers. **Fig. 1** shows an example of an RPM device kit.

OPERATIONAL CONSIDERATIONS

The operational component of an RPM program addresses program management. Although technology allows the capture of health-related data, the data need to be managed in order to improve patient care. The operations team processes the data received. Creating standard workflows that are efficient and support staff working at their fullest potential and top of license are the key for reviewing actionable data. Other areas of focus include program design, device deployment/recovery, and outlining key performance indicators. Incorporating a device deployment and recovery plan that is easy for patients and works within human and financial limitations is essential. Outlining key performance indicators that align with program goals will help measure the program's success and identify areas in need of improvement as the program evolves.

RPM programs can be implemented using internal resources or by outsourcing services to a third party. Decisions about which services might be supported internally or by outsourcing can be tailored to available internal resources and intended goals. A variety of services can be outsourced in an RPM program. These services include the deployment of devices and training of proper device use, monitoring and validating of clinical data, software algorithms for alerting data/decision support, patient interventions, and the return of devices. Even hybrid models have supported program success. These decisions are based on human and material resources and ultimate goals of the program. Many vendors currently provide these services and are very competitive.

Remote Patient Monitoring Team Workflows

Defining program workflows that are standard and support the stated goals are essential and should address patient enrollment, monitoring management, and graduation.

Patient enrollment
  Workflows that accurately identify and efficiently enroll patients into the program are crucial. Clear program inclusion and exclusion criteria are necessary to ensure the right patient population is targeted. These criteria are based on

clinical condition and should be tied to achieving the program's goals. Depending on the program design, referrals could be placed by members of the patient's care team, via automated clinical pathways, or both. An important metric is the time between referral and the full onboarding of the patient into the program. Important components of the onboarding process include patient expectations for testing and program duration, device deployment and training, and patient education on what to do in the event of an emergent situation. Obtaining patient consent and identifying a supervising provider for monitoring is needed for billing compliance.

Monitoring management

The role of the telehealth nurse has expanded as patient care is increasingly shifting from the acute care setting back into the community.[3] Telehealth nurses frequently use technology to engage patients in innovative ways, which may include RPM. RPM nurses may use a variety of tools to engage with patients, including video, telephone, or secure text. This setting allows the nurse to provide health-related education, symptom management, and medication review in a manner that is convenient to the patient. Nurses will be tasked with developing competencies in monitoring biometric data and responding with appropriate interventions.

Telephone triage, secure patient text, and the ability to address emergency situations without face-to-face assessments create unique challenges. Therefore, RPM design should delineate nurse role expectations to meet program goals. For health systems looking to implement RPM, a tiered workforce may prove to be cost-effective. Using roles such as medical assistants or licensed practical nurses (LPNs) in addition to registered nurses (RNs) may assist in creating a centralized team where everyone can practice at the top of licensure. Medical assistants or LPNs play a valuable role in supporting RNs by checking in with patients that are not testing and escalating concerning situations as appropriate.

Key components of effective monitoring include a system to collect and trend the data as well as an alert system to signal abnormal readings. The biometric data will be reviewed by a nurse-led team, who monitor and validate the readings. The development of telehealth technologies should support nurse communication, counseling, coaching, education, and the oversight of care management activity of the remotely monitored patient.

Alert systems need to be actionable for the nursing teams to prioritize and triage. Nurse-led protocols are essential to address emergent scenarios and allow the nursing team to intervene proactively. For example, a patient with heart failure (HF) who has a weight gain of three pounds and shortness of breath or edema may require an intervention. A diuretic protocol would allow the nurse to advise the patient to take an increased dose of their oral diuretic. Protocols such as these allow for autonomous practice on part of the nurse and timely intervention that does not require waiting for a provider response. All protocols connect back to the treating provider for review or continued intervention.

Staffing models for RPM programs can be centralized or decentralized. A centralized nursing model provides data monitoring for many providers. A decentralized model provides data monitoring for patients in a single practice or provider.

Recommended nurse–patient staffing ratios will vary depending on the program structure. A typical staffing ratio is one nurse for every 85 to 100 patients[4] but may range from 50 to 500 depending on program design. Nurses can provide data monitoring, conduct nursing assessments, provide patient education, and escalate validated actionable data to a provider. Non-licensed staff can support the nursing team by validating alerts, troubleshooting devices, and providing calls to patients who are non-adherent.

Patient Case Example: (*This is a fictional example to demonstrate how RPM can improve patient outcomes.*) Mr Smith is an 85-year-old man with a diagnosis of HF who was recently hospitalized for an acute exacerbation. As part of his discharge plan, he was enrolled into an RPM program and provided a scale, blood pressure monitor, and a cellular modem to transmit his daily readings. His at-home diuretic medication dosing was adjusted, whereas he was in the hospital. On his second day of monitoring, his weight increased by 3 pounds since the previous day. The telehealth RN outreached to the patient to review his weight gain and evaluate if he was having any symptoms, such as ankle/abdominal swelling or shortness of breath. The RN confirmed his medications to ensure appropriate use and reviewed the foods he had eaten in the previous 24 hours. The patient admitted to having ankle swelling and shortness of breath after climbing 1 flight of stairs. He also admitted to having lunch with a friend at a local restaurant and eating the chicken noodle soup special. Having a protocol in place that allows the RN to advise the patient to take an additional dose of his diuretic, the RN advised him to do so and then notified the cardiologist of the patient's status. The RN also reiterated the need to adhere to a low-salt diet.

Program graduation

Setting guidelines for length of program enrollment and graduation are crucial to the implementation of a successful program. On enrollment, the patient and/or the caregiver need to be made aware of these guidelines. Maintaining safe staffing ratios is crucial for the program to continue to deliver high-quality patient care. It is important to set graduation criteria to create autonomy for the nursing teams to know when to discharge patients from the program. Graduation criteria can include stability of vitals, noncompliance with testing, achievement of goals, and ability to self-manage condition. Inpatient or ED utilization can also serve as measurable criteria to end monitoring. A crucial part of the graduation process is to ensure the patient is appropriately linked to community-based resources if warranted. A process for managing the devices on graduation is also necessary.

Patient Case Example (*Continued*): Mr Smith continued working with the RPM team for an additional 90 days. During those 90 days, he did not return to the hospital and demonstrated successful management at home. His weights were stable, and he was able to verbalize understanding of low-sodium food choices. He demonstrated that he clearly understood his medication regimen. The RN assessed his readiness for program graduation, and the patient expressed that he was comfortable managing his chronic condition. He was provided with information on how to reenroll if needed and was allowed to keep all the equipment except the modem to continue daily testing independently.

Clinical Considerations: Common Clinical Remote Patient Monitoring Use Cases

As organizations continue to look for innovative solutions to care for patients with respect to value-based payment, RPM programs offer solutions that help drive quality outcomes. CMSs creation of financial incentives has made it easier for health care systems to dedicate time and resources toward targeted patient care. The technological, operational, and financial considerations discussed provide a generalized framework.

RPM programs can support a variety of chronic conditions such as HF, chronic obstructive pulmonary disease (COPD), and diabetes.[2,5–10] Acute or self-limited conditions may also benefit and can include COVID-19, postoperative recovery, and high-risk pregnancy.[11,12] With this information, treatment plans can be personalized based on health data received during monitoring.

According to CMS, 68% of beneficiaries have two or more chronic conditions.[13] These chronic conditions result in significant morbidity and mortality. From a patient perspective, these conditions often result in an inferior quality of life and higher mortality.[14] From a system standpoint, these chronic conditions are responsible for driving most health care expenditures.[15] **Fig. 2** shows many of the common RPM applications aimed at improving care for patients with chronic and acute/self-limiting conditions.

RPM is increasingly being used to care for patients with various acute conditions. The COVID-19 pandemic accelerated this trend, as RPM facilitates access to care especially when face-to-face encounters are not feasible. In part, this led CMS to expand RPM coverage to include acute conditions such as COVID-19 in 2020.[16] The list of potential conditions appropriate for RPM is endless. Much work is ongoing to develop new strategies for monitoring a variety of conditions including but not limited to dementia, stroke, depression, bipolar disorder, and so forth. Applications for RPM are being developed to monitor patients post-surgery to assure appropriate recovery and minimize complications. Several RPM technologies target lifestyle modifications including smoking cessation, diet/exercise, weight loss, and other health coaching designed to improve overall health and sense of well-being.

This section presents a review of common applications currently in practice, including:

1. HF
2. COPD
3. Diabetes

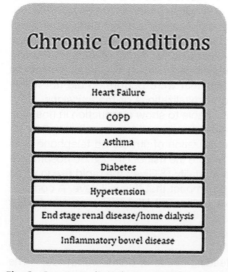
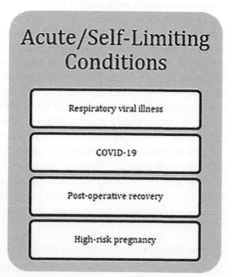

Fig. 2. Common clinical use cases for remote patient monitoring.

4. Respiratory viral illness (COVID-19)

Heart Failure

HF continues to pose a significant medical burden in the United States. In the late 2000s, automatic remote monitoring of cardiac implantable electronic devices was used for the early detection of ventricular arrhythmias as well as device performance. HF is the most frequent cause of readmissions,[8] which consumes a major portion of total dollars spent on HF in the United States.

A straightforward approach to RPM for patients with HF includes a scale so patients can record weight daily. This strategy for monitoring, when successfully executed, can lead to a reduction in HF readmissions. Given the reliance on patients to weigh themselves daily, attempts to improve adherence rates to self-monitoring have included health care team reminders for patients. The Telemonitoring to Improve HF trial sought to compare standard care versus telemonitoring to reduce readmissions.[17] The primary end point was not met despite the additional service of frequent phone-based interactions with patients.[17] A similar outcome was seen in the Telemedical Interventional Monitoring in HF (TIM-HF) trial.[18] There were no differences in all-cause death, cardiovascular death, or HF hospitalizations for telemonitoring of weight and blood pressures.[18]

RPM data collection during the TIM-HF trial included:

- Basic vitals: Blood pressure, oxygen saturation, heart rate, respiratory rate
- Electrocardiogram transmission
- Medication adherence
- Additional data sources such as activity level and daily symptom score[18]

In the TIM-HF trial, the benefits of telemonitoring were observed as part of a multi-component home system with daily wireless transmission of weight, blood pressure, heart rate, heart rhythm, oxygen saturation, and self-rated health status. HF education and structured telephone calls were part of driving success with compliance (97% of patients were 70% compliant).[18] This led to a decline in unplanned cardiovascular hospitalizations and all-cause mortality.[19]

Some concerns with weight monitoring as suggested above are that despite being highly specific for worsening HF, it may not be sensitive enough. The development of weight gain in acute HF exacerbations likely occurs too late to affect therapeutic interventions that would avoid hospitalization or readmission. Bioimpedance, the property of tissues to conduct an electrical signal, can be an earlier signal of decompensating HF. Much of the utilization of bioimpedance has been through implantable electrical devices as mentioned above. The clinical trials that were performed did not follow the impact of impedance values on reduced hospitalizations or readmissions. Similarly, the Diagnostic Outcome Trial in HF was unable to show a reduction in hospitalizations for HF exacerbation when using intrathoracic impedance monitoring.[8]

Further evidence continues to support the utilization of structured telephone calls and telemonitoring as effective measures to reduce the risk of HF-related hospitalizations as well as reducing the risk of all-cause mortality.[20] Given the rapid rise in video integration in virtual visits, it is not yet clear the impact that this will have. A comprehensive multimodal program, as comparable to the TIM-HF2 trial, warrants further consideration for the HF population.

Chronic Obstructive Pulmonary Disease

COPD is a chronic disease and the fourth leading cause of death worldwide.[21] The typical patient with COPD has chronic respiratory symptoms with intervening periods of deterioration known as acute exacerbations. These COPD exacerbations result in a considerable decline in clinical status and an increase in the cost of care. COPD exacerbations are associated with worsening quality of life, increased breathlessness, increased hospitalizations, and increased mortality.[21] Being able to prevent an exacerbation of COPD should translate into considerable clinical and financial benefits. There are clinical strategies, including early antibiotics, steroids, and bronchodilators, which can minimize or eliminate the adverse consequences of COPD exacerbations. It is widely believed that early initiation of these treatments is essential, especially in patients with more advanced disease.

Common biometrics collected in COPD RPM programs:

- Basic vitals: oxygen saturation, heart rate, respiratory rate, and temperature
- Lung capacity: peak flows/spirometry
- Medication adherence
- Additional data sources: air quality, activity level, and daily symptom score[7]

In addition to the collected data, engagement within the program offers opportunities for nurses to provide structured education to COPD patients and caregivers. This education can include understanding disease symptoms, diet, exercise, medication use, pursed-lip breathing, and pulmonary rehabilitation.

Given that acute COPD exacerbations drive utilization and health care costs, there is potential financial benefit to offering RPM as an innovative strategy that can allow for the early detection of decompensation. The clinical potential for RPM includes a reduction in mortality and hospitalization. One systematic review of nine articles suggested that home telemonitoring could reduce COPD exacerbations, reduce hospitalizations for COPD, and improve quality of life in patients with COPD.[7]

Unfortunately, there is not a single factor that equates to COPD deterioration, and it remains unclear how to detect an acute exacerbation early enough to intervene. A typical acute exacerbation of COPD results in a constellation of abnormalities. Other chronic conditions usually have a more direct measure of deterioration, such as elevated glucose in diabetes or a weight gain in HF. Many centers are working to develop composite measures that include both subjective and objective data. One recent study showed concordance with decreased forced expiratory volume (FEV1) and forced vital capacity (FVC), increased use of short-acting bronchodilators, and decreased oxygen saturation with acute exacerbations of COPD.[22]

Diabetes

Another trend in the use of RPM services has been the telemonitoring of diabetes. The United States spends over $327 billion annually on direct and indirect costs of diabetes care, despite a higher prevalence and poorer outcomes compared with other nations worldwide.[23] The social determinants of health, in particular rural living, health literacy, financial constraints, and education level, interfere with the ability to adequately manage chronic illnesses such as diabetes.[24]

RPM data collection usually associated with diabetes includes:

- Blood glucose measurement
- Hemoglobin A1C (HbA1c)
- Additional data sources such as hypoglycemic and hyperglycemic event management[5,6]

Several studies demonstrated the effectiveness of RPM to reduce HbA1c levels. Participants are provided with a blood glucose monitoring device and supplies.

Some devices have a SIM card that can allow direct data transmission to an online platform securely, obviating the need for Internet connections or data plans. In one RPM study, there was sustained reduction in HbA1c at 12 months.[5] Other studies reveal that predominantly rural and low-income populations can achieve HbA1c reductions with RPM for blood glucose readings.[5] Telemedicine for diabetes has proven to be cost-effective as reductions in costs are reflected by a decrease in frequency of hospitalizations and shorter lengths of stay for those participating.[25]

RPM programs that include a comprehensive approach to remote diabetic care have noted that strategies to increase patient engagement along with measurement can have a prolonged impact on HbA1c. One study found that as patient activation increased, the HbA1c achieved after the program decreased.[6] The percentage of patients with HbA1c values of greater than 9% decreased from 20% at baseline to 10.6% at the completion of the program.[6] Engagement tactics included nurse coaches providing medication adherence assessment, nutritional counseling, weight management, and disease self-management support.[6] There was a negative association between patient data uploads and HbA1c at the completion of the program.[6]

Respiratory Viral Illness and COVID-19

COVID-19 has transformed the way clinicians and health systems address treatment of specific disease processes. Specifically, containment efforts during the pandemic focused on the utilization of RPM services to care for hemodynamically stable patients in a non-acute environment. Pulse oximetry has played an increasingly important role in remotely monitoring pulmonary diseases. Oxygen saturation has become a valuable data point in the clinical remote evaluation of patients at risk of respiratory compromise and is core to any remote monitoring program for respiratory illness.

In one such program, patients were referred to the COVID-19 RPM program by the ED provider based on an established set of enrollment criteria. The patient was provided instructions on follow-up as well as a pulse oximeter and thermometer before leaving the ED. Automated emails were subsequently sent to the patient as a prompt to complete the engagement survey about the patient's symptoms and measurements. For patients without a positive response, a tiered escalation model was developed to ensure appropriate triage of the patient symptoms. Fifty-six percent of patients triggering a red flag that required provider evaluation were able to take part in a telehealth visit, avoiding unnecessary exposure and reducing the use of personal protective equipment.

Such RPM programs for COVID became increasingly common during the COVID-19 pandemic. Most programs had a similar structure as above with common enrollment criteria, device monitoring, measurement tracking, and specific escalation criteria to capture a decline in clinical status.[11] For patients requiring escalations in care, additional care options were provided based on provider evaluations. Supervised at-home care could be established for patients as well as a specialist referral (telehealth or live). If necessary, transition to the acute care setting could be arranged.[12]

FINANCIAL CONSIDERATIONS

RPM implementation can be costly when considering the financial requirements to hire and train a clinical team along with purchasing devices. In 2019, CMS began reimbursing for RPM under the Medicare Physician Fee Schedule. CMS has identified five CPT codes that can be billed for RPM services.[26] Beginning in January 2022, additional codes will be made available for remote therapeutic monitoring (RTM). These

Table 1 Remote patient monitoring billing codes	
Code	**Description**
99453	The initial equipment setup for the patient, along with any education on how to use the equipment
99454	The transmission of data every 30 d
99091	The review of data by a qualified health care professional, who spent a minimum of 30 min of time reviewing data, once every 30 d
99457	Initial 20 min of interactive communication between the patient or caregiver and the qualified health care professional
99458	Each additional 20 min of interactive communication between the patient or caregiver and the qualified health care professional

Data from BioIntelliSense. Providing and billing Medicare for remote patient monitoring and treatment management. Accessed: February 2021. https://biointellisense.com/assets/providing-and-billing-medicare-for-remote-patient-monitoring.pdf?v=2.

codes (98975, 98976, 98977, 98980, and 98981) will complement the existing RPM codes. RTM codes will allow for patient self-reported data and the ability for physical therapists or nurses to bill for services.[27]

Table 1 provides a brief description of the RPM billing codes. To bill for RPM, the devices used need to be reliable, valid, and defined as medical devices by Section 201(h) of the FDA.[26] The collection of data must also be electronically transmitted. These codes cannot be billed to patients self-entering their data.

SUMMARY

Despite the interest in and the number of active RPM programs, there is still a paucity of evidence to support the effectiveness of this strategy. The value of RPM to detect early deterioration and result in improved clinical outcomes and decreased health care costs is yet to be proven. Further research needs to be conducted to define the optimal program characteristics and patient population that will benefit most. Continued advancement, including research in the quality and reliability of consumer grade devices, and in the use of predictive analytics to identify deteriorating patients more readily will be critical for the future success of RPM programs.

Many see RPM as an effective tool to better manage patients that are in value-based arrangements. Certainly, technological advances also contribute to easier access to patient health-related data. Clinicians, caregivers, payors, policymakers, and patients alike are working to develop strategies for improving chronic care, and RPM is expected to grow. Future research into RPM programs needs to assess the impact of these programs in alignment with other readmission reduction strategies, such as transition of care, care management, palliative medicine, and rehabilitation services. More detailed financial analysis needs to be included as a part of research efforts to help drive evidence-based health policy and billing decisions.

CLINICS CARE POINTS

- Remote patient monitoring (RPM) services can be structured in a variety of ways to achieve clinical and quality outcomes for populations.
- Telehealth nurses play an integral role in the RPM infrastructure.

- RPM can support clinical and quality outcomes to help patients manage chronic or acute/self-limited conditions.
- Using RPM for patients with heart failure (HF) may reduce HF-related hospital stays and all-cause mortality.
- Using RPM for patients with COPD may reduce exacerbations and hospitalization and improve quality of life.
- In patients with diabetes, RPM may drive increased patient engagement and has a positive impact on HbA1C.
- RPM has assisted organizations to better manage resources in the midst of the COVID-19 pandemic, where hospital beds and health care resources were stretched.
- The availability of the RPM billing codes has created a financial incentive to use these programs.
- Easy-to-use RPM devices, which can be interfaced directly to EMRs, play a key role in program adoption.

DISCLOSURE

The authors have nothing to disclose.

REFERENCES

1. Lacktman NM, Ferrante TB, Goodman RB. 2021 Medicare remote patient monitoring FAQs: CMS issues final rule. Health Care Law Today. 2020. Available at: https://www.foley.com/en/insights/publications/2020/12/2021-remote-patient-monitoring-cms-final-rule. Accessed December 23, 2021.
2. Farias FAC, Dagostini CM, Bicca YA, et al. Remote patient monitoring: A systematic review. Telemed J E Health 2020;26(5):576–83.
3.. Rutledge CM, Gustin T. Preparing nurses for roles in telehealth: Now is the time! OJIN 2021;26(1). https://ojin.nursingworld.org/MainMenuCategories/ANAMarketplace/ANAPeriodicals/OJIN/TableofContents/Vol-26-2021/No1-Jan-2021/Preparing-Nurses-for-Roles-in-Telehealth-Now-is-the-Time.html.
4. Mid-Atlantic Telehealth Resource Center. Remote patient monitoring (RPM) toolkit. Available at: https://www.matrc.org/wp-content/uploads/2019/09/ACFrOgAZizRQ3oro_iD9OoBp9GrOvXRY_sSudMMnn26bNFPfBq8Pij1saJ4ZkbY0tzsfPDnqLmzNENJpvnIYMFQUMZKGHFmG77pWea5prJkm3rTDJwJnYgeC5vz7k6M.pdf. Accessed November 2021.
5. Kirkland EB, Marsden J, Zhang J, et al. Remote patient monitoring sustains reductions of hemoglobin A1c in underserved patients to 12 months. Prim Care Diabetes 2021;15(3):459–63.
6. Su D, Michaud TL, Estabrooks P, et al. Diabetes management through remote patient monitoring: The importance of patient activation and engagement with the technology. Telemed J E Health 2019;25(10):953–9.
7. Cruz J, Brooks D, Marques A. Home telemonitoring effectiveness in COPD: A systematic review. Int J Clin Pract 2014;68(3):369–78.
8. Emani S. Remote monitoring to reduce heart failure readmissions. Curr Heart Fail Rep 2017;14(1):40–7.
9. Ono M, Varma N. Remote monitoring for chronic disease management: Atrial fibrillation and heart failure. Card Electrophysiol Clin 2018;10(1):43–58.
10. O'Reilly JF, Williams AE, Rice I. Health status impairment and costs associated with COPD exacerbation managed in hospital. Int J Clin Pract 2007;61:1112–20.

11. Aalam AA, Hood C, Donelan C, et al. Remote patient monitoring for ED discharges in the COVID-19 pandemic. Emerg Med J 2021;38(3):229–31.
12. Tabacof L, Kellner C, Breyman E, et al. Remote patient monitoring for home management of coronavirus disease 2019 in New York: A cross-sectional observational study. Telemed J E Health 2021;27(6):641–8.
13. Centers for Medicare and Medicaid Services. Chronic conditions overview. Available at: https://www.cms.gov/Research-Statistics-Data-and-Systems/Statistics-Trends-and-Reports/Chronic-Conditions. Accessed December 23, 2021.
14. World Health Organization. Global health estimates: Life expectancy and leading causes of death and disability. Available at: https://www.who.int/data/gho/data/themes/mortality-and-global-health-estimates. Accessed December 2021.
15.. DeVol R, Bedroussian A, Chatterjee A, et al. An unhealthy America: the economic burden of chronic disease-charting a new course to save lives and increase productivity and economic growth. Santa Monica, CA: Milken Institute; 2007.
16. Centers for Medicare and Medicaid Services. Medicare and Medicaid programs: Policy and regulatory revisions in response to the COVID-19 public health emergency. Office of the Federal Register. 2020. Available at: https://www.cms.gov/files/document/covid-final-ifc.pdf. Accessed November 2021.
17. Chaudhry SI, Mattera JA, Curtis JP, et al. Telemonitoring in patients with heart failure. N Engl J Med 2010;363:2301–9.
18. Koehler F, Winkler S, Schieber M, et al. Telemedical interventional monitoring in heart failure (TIM-HF), a randomized, controlled intervention trial investigating the impact of telemedicine on mortality in ambulatory patients with heart failure: study design. Eur J Heart Fail 2010;12(12):1354–62.
19. Koehler F, Koehler K, Deckwart O, et al. Efficacy of telemedical interventional management in patients with heart failure (TIM-HF2): a randomised, controlled, parallel-group, unmasked trial. Lancet 2018;392(10152):1047–57.
20. Conway A, Inglis SC, Clark RA. Effective technologies for noninvasive remote monitoring in heart failure. Telemed J E Health 2014;20(6):531–8.
21. National Center for Chronic Disease Prevention and Health Promotion. COPD. February 22, 2021. Available at: https://www.cdc.gov/copd/index.html. Accessed December 2021.
22. Cooper C, Sirichana W, Arnold M, et al. Remote patient monitoring for the detection of COPD exacerbation. Int J COPD 2020;15:2005–13.
23. Yang W, Dall TM, Beronjia K, et al. Economic costs of diabetes in the U.S. in 2017. Diabetes Care 2018;41(5):917–28.
24. Hill-Briggs F, Adler NE, Berkowitz SA, et al. Social determinants of health and diabetes: A scientific review. Diabetes Care 2021;44(1):258–79.
25. Randall MH, Haulsee ZM, Zhang J, et al. The effect of remote patient monitoring on the primary care clinic visit frequency among adults with type 2 diabetes. Int J Med Inform 2020;143.
26. BioIntelliSense. Providing and billing medicare for remote patient monitoring and treatment management. 2021. Available at: https://biointellisense.com/assets/providing-and-billing-medicare-for-remote-patient-monitoring.pdf?v=2. Accessed December 2021.
27. Lacktman NM, Ferrante TB. CMS proposes new remote therapeutic monitoring codes: What you need to know. Health Care Law Today. Published July 15, 2021. Available at: https://www.foley.com/en/insights/publications/2021/07/cms-new-remote-therapeutic-monitoring-codes. Accessed December 2021.

Virtual Access to Subspecialty Care

Matthew B. Mackwood, MD, MPH[a], Ameet S. Nagpal, MD, MS, MEd, MBA[b],
Joyce Yuen, DO[c], Ramon S. Cancino, MD, MBA, MS[c],*

KEYWORDS

- Telehealth • Telemedicine • Virtual • Access • Subspecialty care

KEY POINTS

- Before the public health emergency, many subspecialties have a long history of telehealth innovation.
- Telehealth has been demonstrated to improve access and patient satisfaction while, in many cases, maintaining high-quality outcomes of in-person appointments.
- There is much motivation to increase access to telehealth but this effort must be done while monitoring equal access of these services for all and maintenance or improvement in the value of care.
- National regulations have the potential to drive innovations, which would benefit all.
- Primary care physicians could partner with subspecialists to develop processes to link patients to the right subspecialist at the right time and in the right visit type.

INTRODUCTION

Recent expansion in both payment and need for telehealth across all areas of health care has the potential to bring both health-care innovation and patient access to improve health outcomes. With this expansion have come changes in access to subspecialty providers. This article reviews the history and current state of telehealth access in many areas of subspecialty care.

TELEHEALTH MODALITIES

There are several separate but complementary approaches to leveraging telehealth services for outpatient care: (1) the direct provision of care to patients via telehealth (reviewed at more length by specialty below), (2) provider-to-provider-to-patient

[a] Department of Community and Family Medicine, Geisel School of Medicine, DHMC, One Medical Center Drive, Lebanon, NH 03756, USA; [b] Department of Orthopaedics & Physical Medicine, Medical University of South Carolina, Clinical Sciences Building, CSB, 96 Jonathan Lucas Street, MSC Code: 708, Charleston, SC 29425, USA; [c] Department of Family & Community Medicine, Joe R & Teresa Lozano Long School of Medicine, UT Health San Antonio, 7703 Floyd Curl Drive, MC 7843, San Antonio, TX 78229, USA
* Corresponding author.
E-mail address: cancinor@uthscsa.edu

Prim Care Clin Office Pract 49 (2022) 557–573
https://doi.org/10.1016/j.pop.2022.05.001
0095-4543/22/© 2022 Elsevier Inc. All rights reserved.

primarycare.theclinics.com

communication via telehealth in real-time during a clinical encounter (not well-studied in an outpatient context, in contrast to, eg, inpatient tele-intensive care), and (3) asynchronous provider-to-provider communication separate from a direct patient encounter.

Asynchronous Provider-To-Provider Consultation

Project extension for community healthcare outcomes

Project Extension for Community Healthcare Outcomes (ECHO) is a model where a clinical specialist or team of specialists provides longitudinal support to primary care clinicians through group reviews of the latest evidence and focused patient case discussions.[1–3] Project ECHO was originally deployed to provide remote education on Hepatitis C virus (HCV) management. In that context, community practitioners (meeting via teleconference) presented cases on HCV-positive patients; discussed relevant details including history, comorbid illness or issues, and physical examination and laboratory test findings; and described ongoing treatment complications. These cases were then discussed with expert support in hepatology, infectious disease, psychiatry, and substance abuse to both provide specific guidance to the providers as well as highlight general principles in management to support ongoing independent practice.[3] A systematic review in 2017 found that these models tended to enroll wide numbers of providers (ranging from as low as 9 to as high as 710, with a median of 38), produce a high level of provider participant satisfaction, and increase provider knowledge and confidence on prepost assessment.[1] One retrospective analysis of 377 VA patients with uncomplicated HCV showed no difference between primary and specialty care services.[4] Other contexts had more limited data, with one study suggesting Project ECHO training resulted in subsequent improved A1c values in diabetes.[5] The systematic review of the original HCV model found it cost-effective, rating an average savings of $1352 per patient compared with conventional approaches.[1]

E-consults

E-consults have been studied in settings where it has been shown to be minimally disruptive to provider workflows and reduced "inappropriate clinic visits" while increasing necessary follow-up visits for specialties, compared with traditional referral processes.[6–8] This is tempered by findings of variable levels of specialist satisfaction and in reports of overall impressions of increased care quality, underscoring the need for effective implementation, monitoring, and feedback to make optimal use of such systems.[6] Overall impact to access in terms of avoided "unnecessary referrals" is reported in a 2019 systematic review ranging from 7.4% to 78% reduction on the extremes and a 22% to 68% range representing most of the studies identified. Such changes in access were generally shown to be cost-effective; across 6 studies in the review, cost savings ranged from $5-$50 per e-consult compared with face-to-face.[7] Typical e-consult turnaround time was 1 to 6 days across 5 studies. Typical specialist time spent to respond was 20, 30, and 78 minutes in 3 separate studies. Referring provider-reported conclusiveness in 2 studies rated 74% to 89%. One study of a system with a mature e-consult implementation reported 3-fold variation in the rate of requests being resolved without a visit after e-consult, from 11.4% to 32.3% across bottom to top decile of provider. Lowest rates of resolution without visit were seen in podiatry, ophthalmology, otolaryngology, and gynecology, with highest rates among hematology/oncology, neurology, cardiology, and rheumatology. In this study, lower rates of e-consultation "first touch resolution" corresponded to lower provider-reported engagement with performing e-consults.[9,15]

Specialty-Specific Reviews

Cardiology

Cardiology consultations via telehealth have included chief complaints such as palpitations, chest pain, dizziness/syncope, dyslipidemia, hypertension, patients with an abnormal electrogram, and patients with a family history of genetic disorders. A 2013 systematic review and meta-analysis of trials on home blood pressure telemonitoring showed significant improvement in blood pressure control relative to usual care.[10] There is less evidence supporting the benefits of telehealth in hypertension management in terms of cost, drug safety, deaths, or hospitalizations.[11] Cardiac rehabilitation programs that used telehealth have shown improved outcomes,[12,13] and a retrospective study of cardiology telehealth visits at an academic pediatric center between 2016 and 2019 showed reduction in cost and travel time for patients and families.[14]

Telehealth in cardiology may use the use of tele echocardiography, remote electrophysiological monitoring and teleausculation.[15] During the COVID-19 pandemic, cardiologists used digital wearables and other at-home monitoring devices to obtain vital signs and electrocardiogram tracings.[11,16] Studies have shown encouraging results of implantable hemodynamic monitoring.[17,18]

There is concern that disparities exist in access to telehealth and medical devices to facilitate virtual visits. Multiple observational studies have shown that patients that are non-White, older, in lower socioeconomic groups, non-English speaking, or with lower education had lower utilization of telehealth and access to cardiac devices to facilitate virtual visits.[19–21]

Dermatology

Because of the expansive work in teledermatology, it is the specialty used the most by remote primary care physicians (PCPs) for telehealth consults as early as 1997.[22] Diagnostic accuracy and treatment effectiveness with teledermatology are equal to in-clinic visits.[23] Teledermatology has also demonstrated reduced in-person referrals to dermatologists and improved access to care,[24] particularly in underserved communities.[25,26] Many studies have been published demonstrating effective processes to implement teledermatology consults in inpatient and outpatient settings.[27–32] This article will highlight the most impactful research in this area.[9]

Reports of accurate diagnosis using telehealth and crossmatching to biopsy range from 60% to 100%.[33] The American Academy of Dermatology (AAD) states that telehealth is equally effective compared with in-person care in the management of inflammatory skin diseases such as atopic dermatitis and psoriasis.[34] In a Spanish study, a cost analysis of teledermatology versus in-person care demonstrated an average savings of 11.4 € per patient visit.[35] In a study of 700 outpatients seen in primary care clinics in Philadelphia and referred for teledermatology consults, researchers demonstrated a 27% decrease in in-person visits and a 3.29% decrease in emergency department visits. The mean expected savings from these changes were estimated as $10.00 to $52.65 per patient.[36] In a retrospective study of more than 2300 referrals from PCPs to dermatologists, e-consults were found to improve access to care for medically underserved populations. In this study, 11% of referrals resulted in a confirmed appointment (median wait time 77 days) before implementation of e-consults. After implementation, 44% of consults were sent via e-consults, and 16% of those required in-person consultation with a median wait time of 28 days.[25] In another study of Medicaid claims data, of patients who received dermatologic care, 48.5% did so via teledermatology. About 75.7% of newly enrolled Medicaid patients who accessed dermatologic care did so via telehealth. Teledermatologists were more likely to care for viral skin lesions and acne (46.7% of visits), whereas in-person dermatologists were more likely to care for psoriasis and skin neoplasms (36.8% of visits) despite the AAD position statement of equal efficacy of treatment of psoriasis in both settings.[26] Data on teledermatology are compelling and show at least equivalency for effectiveness of diagnosis and treatment, decreased cost of care, and increased access to care.

Endocrinology

Telehealth has been used in endocrinology for underserved patient populations that lack access to specialty care due to location.[37–39] It has been found to be safe and associated with time savings, cost savings, and high patient and provider satisfaction.[37,39,40]

Telehealth has been successfully used for new-onset diabetes training and education[41] as well as for patients with an established diabetes diagnosis.[37,40] There seems to be a significant opportunity to achieve better efficiency in diabetes care and self-management with telehealth.[42–44] A meta-analysis supports the use of telehealth in monitoring hemoglobin A1c in type 2 diabetes.[45] There have been reported cases of avoiding diabetic ketoacidosis hospital admissions with the use of telehealth.[46]

Low-risk patients with thyroid disease can receive medication adjustments, medical consultations, or ongoing follow-ups through telehealth.[47]

Gastroenterology

Before the COVID-19 pandemic, the use of telehealth in gastroenterology was ranked second lowest among internal medicine specialties because less than 8% of gastroenterologists used telehealth in their practice, according to a 2016 survey. Telehealth before the pandemic was focused on access to remote or underserved populations. For instance, Project ECHO was initiated in 2003 to provide telementoring for clinicians treating chronic HCV remotely.[48]

Because of the COVID-19 pandemic, providers were forced to scale down in-person visits. A hybrid gastroenterology consultation program trial during a continuous 5-month period during the pandemic at an academic center noted that more than 71% of virtual consults were resolved without a need for a clinic visit.[49] Additionally, a randomized trial showed that patients with inflammatory bowel disease, who had close follow-up with remote technology, had decreased subsequent hospitalizations.[50]

There has been positive patient and clinician experience with telehealth in gastroenterology.[49,51,52] Although the value of telehealth is recognized, the future is uncertain. Provider-perceived telehealth barriers include technical issues and lack of patient preparedness.[53] A survey of gastroenterologists and hepatologists in 2020 revealed that up to 20% plan to completely transition to in-person visits after the COVID-19 pandemic.[53]

Infectious diseases

Telehealth for outpatient infectious diseases has a few areas of predominant focus including management of human immunodeficiency virus (HIV), HCV, and tuberculosis (TB).[54] Each of these conditions share a common feature of requiring nuance in medication selection and monitoring, where ease of access to care may play a key role in long-term adherence, management, and cure/sustained remission.

Human immunodeficiency virus care. Telehealth has been leveraged for decades in HIV care, using remote communication via telephone to preserve patient anonymity in screening and diagnosis.[55] In contemporary HIV care, the use of telehealth to support the safe and effective use of preexposure and postexposure prophylaxis is an area of ongoing study, including the use of Project ECHO and e-consult modalities to encourage management by primary care.[56] Evidence supports the use of telehealth in HIV care to promote follow-up and retention for remote patients along with preserving privacy; however, a relatively high proportion of HIV-positive patients are homeless compared with the general population and telehealth can be challenging to deliver privately in such a context.[57,58] Telehealth use overall showed slightly superior rates of viral suppression compared with in-person care in a cluster randomized VA study of HIV care in Iowa in 2015 to 2016.[59] One observational study in San Francisco noted higher rates of viral loads among patients managed via telehealth during the COVID-19 pandemic despite lower no-show rates and more frequent visits via telehealth in such patients, especially among patients who were homeless, Black, or young (aged less than 35 years), suggesting possible confounders affecting HIV adherence in the pandemic and the potential benefit for "wrap-around" social services in clinic which are relatively less accessible in a telehealth context.[58] Clinical outcome data was limited otherwise, and there is a need for further study of telehealth and its impact on patient care along the HIV care continuum from prevention and diagnosis to chronic care management.[57,60]

Hepatitis C and other applications. HCV is another area of study for telehealth in infectious diseases, with Project ECHO implementation demonstrated to expand access to care.[61] TB has been less studied but has shown promise in facilitating directly observed therapy, a longstanding mainstay in treatment.[54] Travel medicine is another area where telehealth could have promise, potentially enabling GPS-accurate travel history for identifying exposure risks.[62]

Outside of HIV care and HCV, the evidence for the use of telehealth to enable access to outpatient infectious disease care is limited,[63] and cost-efficacy data are lacking.[54] Although telehealth shows great promise for improving access, the relatively higher comorbidity rate of some infectious diseases such as HIV with complicating social determinants and other medical conditions such as substance use disorder lends itself to careful study among vulnerable populations. Future research can help ensure implementation includes holistic support toward improving health, or otherwise runs the risk of undermining any benefit from telehealth's increased access. To that end, increasing support for infectious disease management in a specialist-supported, well-integrated primary care practice model would seem promising.

Neurology

Before the pandemic, teleneurology had been well championed and studied in the use of telehealth in contexts including the rapid evaluation of stroke in emergency settings.[64–66] There has emerged a clear consensus for the potential benefit of telehealth across a variety of conditions.[67]

A 2019 review suggested benefits to outpatient neurology access for the care and management multiple sclerosis, neurooncology, and the management of cerebrovascular disorders and their underlying risk factors such as hypertension and diabetes.[68] Specific technological applications proposed ranged from teleconsulting and remote management to the monitoring and remote control of deep brain stimulation or infusion pumps, leveraging of teleradiology and telepathology to aid diagnosis, and expansion of use cases for telerehabilitation and general outpatient telemetry for the monitoring of biological functions.[68] The use of video is seen as beneficial for variety of neurologic conditions ranging from vertigo to neuromuscular diseases, dementia, and movement disorders such as Parkinson disease.[69] Epilepsy care is an opportunity to expand teleneurology virtual clinics with ambulatory electroencephalogram (EEG) to facilitate access.[70] Routine outpatient headache management is another promising area for teleneurology intervention.[71]

Some examination elements remain barriers to full telehealth adoption, including the effective remote examination of deep tendon reflexes, vestibular function, and the performance of fundoscopy.[67,72] Despite this, in one study of a multisite pediatric neurology department's COVID-19 transition at Children's Hospital of Philadelphia analyzing more than 1200 visits, only 5% of visits were recommended for necessary in-person follow-up and providers considered telehealth satisfactory in 93% of visits.[73] Contrast with a mixed-methods study where more than 700 patients were surveyed and interviewed after being seen by Neurology at Wake Forest, patients frequently perceived telehealth evaluation to be insufficient to fully assess their examination (nearly half of respondents), although more than 75% of patients reported the telehealth visit met their needs without significant differences noted between telephone and video evaluation. Telehealth was viewed as more acceptable for follow-up visits and the care of patients with stable diagnoses by patients in the same study. Patients reported a variety of scenarios where they had an unmet need following a telehealth visit that could have been addressed in person, such as medication injections and delays in paperwork completion. In-person care also remains important for in-person evaluations such as nerve conduction testing.[74] Some of these barriers are potentially able to be addressed with trained telepresenters in some contexts but such approaches remain an area for future study, particularly in a prospective, controlled trial format to gauge the value of video examination for the broad range of neurologic conditions and population settings seen for care.[67]

Ophthalmology

The existing literature base primarily supports the use of models with remote trained examiners obtaining high-quality images for later review (store-and-forward), the most common conditions being diabetic retinopathy and glaucoma screening.[75] Other conditions amenable to teleophthalmology in the literature include macular degeneration, retinopathy of prematurity, and triage of eye conditions (such as in the emergency room). Technologic advances are enabling the use of smartphone-connected autorefraction testing for prescription glasses.[76] These evaluations typically require a significant infrastructure for specialized equipment and training (frequently studied in conjunction with existing primary care or emergency room infrastructure); as such an ideal teleophthalmologic model might best be considered as a "hybrid" where patients still present to a medical site with appropriate setup for examination but are remote from the ophthalmologist until an in-person ophthalmologic examination is deemed necessary.[76,77]

Pain management

Pilot studies and retrospective cohort studies have evaluated the utility of telehealth services for pain management.[78] Integrated care models with primary care using pain management services via telehealth have been described but not studied.[79–81] In one study, military PCPs were given access to video consults with pain management specialists as well as an online pain management curriculum. Patients were asked to assess their pain at various intervals up until 8 weeks after their visit with a PCP. Data are still pending from this study.[79] In a qualitative assessment, 48 e-consults to pain management specialists from PCPs were assessed for the types of patients who were most likely to be referred via this form of consultation. The most common patient diagnoses included chronic pain patients with mental health diagnoses, substance dependence, and social complexity.[80]

In a case series of 54 patients referred for interventional pain procedures who underwent telehealth evaluations, the referral period gradually decreased as the system evolved. No clinical disease progression was noted in between the telehealth evaluation and the procedure for these patients.[82]

An analysis of 16 patients with teleprogramming of spinal cord stimulators demonstrated high levels of success. One hundred percent (4/4) of the physicians thought that patients' needs were addressed appropriately, all patients thought that their pain quickly resolved, and only 1/16 required additional follow-up.[83] At the time of writing of this article, teleprogramming for spinal cord stimulators is not widely available, and this data indicates that in the future patients may be able to access this care more quickly.

A Brazilian retrospective study analyzed the impact of asynchronous telehealth consultations from PCPs to orthopedic surgeons for musculoskeletal complaints (26.1% spine, 16.6% foot, 13.8% knee, and others less than 10%). Of 1174 teleconsultations assessed, only 38.4% of these required evaluation by an orthopedic specialist.[84] Asynchronous consultation by orthopedic surgeons or musculoskeletal specialists may dramatically decrease the necessity for full evaluation from the specialist.

A Veteran's Administration (VA) study on the use of telehealth to treat patients with chronic pain showed the potential for a disparity in care. Veterans in urban settings were less likely to use telehealth services compared with those in rural settings. The researchers expressed concern that patients who live in rural settings may be replacing in-person visits with telehealth visits because of inability to access in-person services, whereas those patients in urban centers continued to use in-person services because of proximity.

A unique study demonstrated no differences in transactional costs between in-person and telehealth visits for chronic pain services.[85]

Palliative and Hospice care
By its nature, most patients cared for by palliative care are at increased risk for COVID-19 exposure, and consultations are often focused on discussion, goals of care, and matters not requiring extensive physical examination or evaluation. Telehealth is efficacious for a variety of applications ranging from education and information sharing to symptom management and decision-making in care.[86,87] Data from the United Kingdom suggest its benefit for providing continuity of care (eg, off-hours telephonic support) in addition to the previously noted applications.[88] Research evaluating outcomes of telehealth as a strategy to expand access or the equitability of access in palliative care is limited and further study is crucial to the field.[86,87]

Hospice care has an evidence base supporting the generally high acceptability of the incorporation of telehealth for patients and caregivers; data on implementation beyond gauging acceptability have not been reported.[89,90]

Physical medicine and rehabilitation
Reports of successful integration of telerehabilitation as a consultation service in the Philippines demonstrated initial success during the COVID-19 pandemic.[91] There have also been reports of success with telerehabilitation in amputee care and patients with acquired brain injury.[92,93] Recommended practice patterns surrounding virtual physical therapy have also been published.[94] Low-quality evidence have

demonstrated that physical therapy and occupational therapy can be used successfully for the following needs: modified evaluations, home exercise programs, group visits, assistive device training, self-care training, home environment assessments, and wheelchair assessments.[94] Lack of evidence of safety and efficacy is one of several reasons that there has been significant concern regarding whether access to telehealth services in the rehabilitation setting may further widen the inequity gap to care in patients with disabilities.[95]

The most robust study in this specialty was performed on patients who had sustained a stroke and had motor deficits in the upper extremity. A total of 124 patients were randomized to either telerehabilitation or in-clinic rehabilitation. Both groups had sustained improvement in upper extremity function and noninferiority of telerehabilitation was statistically significant.[96]

Psychiatry

Between 2010 and 2017, the use of telehealth in psychiatry by state agencies increased from 15.2% to 29.2%.[97] A national survey of emergency departments in 2016 showed that psychiatry was the second most common application of telehealth in the emergency room setting after neurology and stroke consults.[98]

Studies suggest that telehealth broadens access and improves the rate of attainment of behavioral goals.[99,100] At the outpatient psychiatry division at Massachusetts General Hospital, 5% of visits were virtual in March 2019 compared with more than 97% visits in March 2020.[101] Further challenges include the need for more careful safety planning for high-risk patients, maintaining professional boundaries in a relatively informal virtual setting, and continuing care team collaboration without physical locations.[102]

Urology

Before COVID-19, one cross-sectional international survey found 15.8% of urologists used telehealth in clinical practice.[103] A study of a single institution's VA data found that the most common reasons for urologic telehealth referrals were sexual dysfunction (26.8%), lower urinary tract symptoms (20.6%), hematuria (15.0%), prostate cancer (13.3%), and elevated PSA (12.1%).[104] Before the pandemic, the most common telehealth modality was video visits; studies reported a high level of satisfaction and found that they were an effective and safe means of conducting follow-up visits.[105] During COVID-19, one study found that urologists demonstrated the highest use of telehealth visits among surgical specialties during the late pandemic period.[106] Small studies during this time period showed high levels of satisfaction from patients, their families, and providers.[107,108]

A cross-sectional survey of 620 urologists from 58 different countries and 6 continents found that the highest proportion of telehealth visits were for oncology practices followed by nononcology, general, and pediatrics.[103] A small study of a rural patient population found that benefits including convenience were found for pediatric urology patients requiring low-acuity care.[109] Thirty-four percent of the study population indicated they would have driven between 50 and 99 miles for in-person visits, 58% would have lost time at work.

Telehealth services have been successfully implemented in several preoperative and postoperative settings. One study compared video visits to "on site" visits of postoperative pediatric patients and found no surgical complications in either group.[110] A European study of adults found postoperative video visits were associated with equivalent efficiency, similar satisfaction, and significantly lower patient costs when compared with office visits in a randomized group of men with a history of prostate cancer.[111] Similar results were found in a survey of patients and providers who took part in a preoperative and postoperative clinic in Nebraska.[112] In a study of postoperative patients, researchers found that, using a commercially available tablet on postoperative day 1 for telerounding, patients expressed a high level of satisfaction.[113]

In a study of the VA Greater Lost Angeles Healthcare System, researchers found that urology telehealth clinics expanded access to visits for lower urinary tract symptoms (35%), elevated PSA (15%), and prostate cancer (14%).[114]

Challenges

The expansion of virtual care services during the COVID-19 pandemic impacted access to patient care. Among 33.6 million Medicare beneficiaries with a usual source of care who reported that their provider currently offers telehealth appointments, 45% said they had a telehealth visit with a doctor or other health professional between the summer and fall of 2020. Most of these beneficiaries (56%) reported accessing care using telephone visits while a smaller proportion reported video (28%) or both video and telephone (16%).[115] In addition, specialty use of telehealth expanded although there were differences in implementation. Use of virtual care services ranged from 9% of ophthalmologists to 68% of endocrinologists.[116]

It remains to be seen how telehealth will continue as the public health crisis improves. Patients and providers may prefer the comfort of an in-person consultation, and evidence needs to be more robust to reinforce any policies or approaches that champion direct telehealth access to specialty providers as a default. This is especially true with regard to evaluating the differences in care quality and outcomes between telephone and video care; the use of video is clearly favored by certain populations, and policy decisions for differential reimbursement or emphasis on video risk leaving behind many in the digital divide.[117]

Other factors may affect the ability of patients to access telehealth care. A study of patients at a single academic institution being seen for urologic conditions in 2020 found that, although there were no differences in telehealth utilization after stratifying providers by age, sex, or training type (physician or advanced practice provider), patients who were Hispanic, older, or had Medicaid insurance were significantly less likely to access telehealth during the pandemic.[118]

It remains to be seen if telehealth visits bring true value to health care in every specialty. One study found that care initially beginning via a telehealth appointment more frequently generated related visits within a 30-day period.[119] This could be a signal of either increased health care utilization or could reflect expanded access to care.

Opportunities

COVID-19 has accelerated the growth of telehealth as a consultative service across many specialties. Dermatology was uniquely ahead of other specialties in their usage of telehealth, with other specialties now following suit. Given that teledermatology has demonstrated equal effectiveness for many conditions, the future of this field may lie in moving to exclusive telehealth models, in which PCPs can send "store and forward" images to dermatologists, whose practices may come to resemble that of radiologists.

For other specialties, the use of telehealth has allowed for improved access, which will only improve further with enhanced models of delivery of care. Because the Centers for Medicare and Medicaid Services (CMS) have recently codified a long-term structure for payment for telehealth services, specialists will feel comfortable establishing teleconsultation relationships with PCPs.[120] Although there are regulations surrounding the use of telehealth consultation in the new CMS fee schedules that may delay access, this article has demonstrated that access is typically enhanced by the use of telehealth. There is cost savings associated with the use of telehealth, and this may drive future implementation.

Continued expansion of provider-to-provider telehealth look promising and are worth continued study. Such work should extend beyond the existing literature to focus on patient-oriented outcome evidence on which policy decisions can soundly rest. Telehealth increases the ease with which patients can be reached and engaged for ongoing care management and is generally seen as appropriate for follow-up care of many conditions. Continued study of the benefits of direct patient visits for telehealth for access, particularly among complex and historically underserved populations, will help to provide a clear road map to improving the equitability as well as the quality of medical care.

SUMMARY

Subspecialty telehealth care is an expanding field that has brought multiple benefits to patients, and there is much interest to examine other possibilities. Because technology has caught up to subspecialist and patient needs, the benefits include increased access, maintained quality of care, and improved patient experience. There is also a recognition of the limitations of telehealth. Patient and provider technological or social determinants limitations, lack of physical examination, cost of implementation, and questions about future payments affect widespread dissemination. Therefore, the benefits of telehealth to subspecialty care are often balanced by the multiple risks. Nevertheless, there is broad momentum to move the needle forward in subspecialty telehealth to help patients.

PCPs may be unaware of the telehealth services and options local subspecialists offer. To best serve patients, PCPs could partner with subspecialists to develop processes to link patients to the right subspecialist at the right time and in the right visit type.

DISCLOSURE

The authors declare that they have no relevant or material financial interests that relate to the research described in this article.

REFERENCES

1. Zhou C, Crawford A, Serhal E, et al. The impact of project ECHO on participant and patient outcomes: a systematic review. Acad Med 2016;91(10):1439–61.

2. McBain RK, Sousa JL, Rose AJ, et al. Impact of project ECHO models of medical tele-education: a systematic review. J Gen Intern Med 2019;34(12): 2842–57.

3. Arora S, Geppert CMA, Kalishman S, et al. Academic health center management of chronic diseases through knowledge networks: Project ECHO. Acad Med J Assoc Am Med Coll 2007;82(2):154–60.

4. Syed TA, Bashir MH, Farooqui SM, et al. Treatment outcomes of hepatitis c-infected patients in specialty clinic vs. primary care physician clinic: a comparative analysis. Gastroenterol Res Pract 2019;2019:8434602.

5. Watts SA, Roush L, Julius M, et al. Improved glycemic control in veterans with poorly controlled diabetes mellitus using a specialty care access network-extension for community healthcare outcomes model at primary care clinics. J Telemed Telecare 2016;22(4):221–4.

6. Vimalananda VG, Gupte G, Seraj SM, et al. Electronic consultations (e-consults) to improve access to specialty care: a systematic review and narrative synthesis. J Telemed Telecare 2015;21(6):323–30.

7. Liddy C, Moroz I, Mihan A, et al. A systematic review of asynchronous, provider-to-provider, electronic consultation services to improve access to specialty care available worldwide. Telemed J E-Health 2019;25(3):184–98.

8. Liddy C, Drosinis P, Keely E. Electronic consultation systems: worldwide prevalence and their impact on patient care-a systematic review. Fam Pract 2016; 33(3):274–85.

9. Barnett ML, Yee HF, Mehrotra A, et al. Los Angeles safety-net program econsult system was rapidly adopted and decreased wait times to see specialists. Health Aff Proj Hope 2017;36(3):492–9.

10. Omboni S, Gazzola T, Carabelli G, et al. Clinical usefulness and cost effectiveness of home blood pressure telemonitoring: meta-analysis of randomized controlled studies. J Hypertens 2013;31(3):455–67, discussion 467-468.

11. Omboni S, McManus RJ, Bosworth HB, et al. Evidence and recommendations on the use of telemedicine for the management of arterial hypertension: an international expert position paper. Hypertens Dallas Tex 1979 2020;76(5):1368–83.

12. Bostrom J, Sweeney G, Whiteson J, et al. Mobile health and cardiac rehabilitation in older adults. Clin Cardiol 2020;43(2):118–26.

13. Thamman R, Janardhanan R. Cardiac rehabilitation using telemedicine: the need for tele cardiac rehabilitation. Rev Cardiovasc Med 2020;21(4):497–500.

14. Phillips AA, Sable CA, Atabaki SM, et al. Ambulatory cardiology telemedicine: a large academic pediatric center experience. J Investig Med 2021;69(7):1372–6.

15. Satou GM, Rheuban K, Alverson D, et al. American heart association congenital cardiac disease committee of the council on cardiovascular disease in the young and council on quality care and outcomes research. telemedicine in pediatric cardiology: a scientific statement from the American heart association. Circulation 2017;135(11):e648–78.

16. Lakkireddy DR, Chung MK, Gopinathannair R, et al. Guidance for cardiac electrophysiology during the COVID-19 pandemic from the heart rhythm society COVID-19 Task force; electrophysiology section of the American college of cardiology; and the electrocardiography and arrhythmias committee of the council on clinical cardiology, American heart association. Heart Rhythm 2020;17(9): e233–41.

17. Almufleh A, Ahluwalia M, Givertz MM, et al. Short-term outcomes in ambulatory heart failure during the COVID-19 pandemic: insights from pulmonary artery pressure monitoring. J Card Fail 2020;26(7):633–4.

18. Oliveros E, Mahmood K, Mitter S, et al. Pulmonary artery pressure monitoring during the COVID-19 pandemic in New York city. J Card Fail 2020;26(10):900–1.

19. Krishnaswami A, Beavers C, Dorsch MP, et al. Innovations, cardiovascular team and the geriatric cardiology councils, American College of cardiology. gerotechnology for older adults with cardiovascular diseases: JACC state-of-the-art review. J Am Coll Cardiol 2020;76(22):2650–70.

20. Wang X, Hidrue MK, Del Carmen MG, et al. Sociodemographic disparities in outpatient cardiology telemedicine during the COVID-19 pandemic. Circ Cardiovasc Qual Outcomes 2021;14(8):e007813.

21. Haynes N, Ezekwesili A, Nunes K, et al. Can you see my screen?" addressing racial and ethnic disparities in telehealth. Curr Cardiovasc Risk Rep 2021; 15(12):23.

22. Norton SA, Burdick AE, Phillips CM, et al. Teledermatology and underserved populations. Arch Dermatol 1997;133(2):197–200.
23. Lee JJ, English JC. Teledermatology: a review and update. Am J Clin Dermatol 2018;19(2):253–60.
24. Giavina-Bianchi M, Santos AP, Cordioli E. Teledermatology reduces dermatology referrals and improves access to specialists. EClinicalMedicine 2020; 29-30:100641.
25. Naka F, Lu J, Porto A, et al. Impact of dermatology eConsults on access to care and skin cancer screening in underserved populations: A model for teledermatology services in community health centers. J Am Acad Dermatol 2018;78(2): 293–302.
26. Uscher-Pines L, Malsberger R, Burgette L, et al. Effect of teledermatology on access to dermatology care among medicaid enrollees. JAMA Dermatol 2016; 152(8):905–12.
27. Dhaduk K, Miller D, Schliftman A, et al. Implementing and optimizing inpatient access to dermatology consultations via telemedicine: an experiential study. Telemed J E-health Off J Am Telemed Assoc 2021;27(1):68–73.
28. Wang RF, Trinidad J, Lawrence J, et al. Improved patient access and outcomes with the integration of an eConsult program (teledermatology) within a large academic medical center. J Am Acad Dermatol 2020;83(6):1633–8.
29. Costello CM, Cumsky HJL, Maly CJ, et al. Improving access to care through the establishment of a local, teledermatology network. Telemed J E-health Off J Am Telemed Assoc 2020;26(7):935–40.
30. Coustasse A, Sarkar R, Abodunde B, et al. Use of teledermatology to improve dermatological access in rural areas. Telemed J E-health Off J Am Telemed Assoc 2019;25(11):1022–32.
31. Sharma P, Kovarik CL, Lipoff JB. Teledermatology as a means to improve access to inpatient dermatology care. J Telemed Telecare 2016;22(5):304–10.
32. Raugi GJ, Nelson W, Miethke M, et al. Teledermatology implementation in a VHA secondary treatment facility improves access to face-to-face care. Telemed J E-health Off J Am Telemed Assoc 2016;22(1):12–7.
33. Wang RH, Barbieri JS, Nguyen HP, et al. Group for Research of policy dynamics in dermatology. clinical effectiveness and cost-effectiveness of teledermatology: where are we now, and what are the barriers to adoption? J Am Acad Dermatol 2020;83(1):299–307.
34. American Academy of Dermatology Association. Position statement on teledermatology. 2021. Available at: https://server.aad.org/Forms/Policies/Uploads/PS/PS-Teledermatology.pdf?. Accessed January 15, 2022.
35. Vidal-Alaball J, Garcia Domingo JL, Garcia Cuyàs F, et al. A cost savings analysis of asynchronous teledermatology compared to face-to-face dermatology in Catalonia. BMC Health Serv Res 2018;18(1):650.
36. Yang X, Barbieri JS, Kovarik CL. Cost analysis of a store-and-forward teledermatology consult system in Philadelphia. J Am Acad Dermatol 2019;81(3):758–64.
37. Xu T, Pujara S, Sutton S, et al. Telemedicine in the management of type 1 diabetes. Prev Chronic Dis 2018;15:E13.
38. Balamurugan A, Hall-Barrow J, Blevins MA, et al. A pilot study of diabetes education via telemedicine in a rural underserved community–opportunities and challenges: a continuous quality improvement process. Diabetes Educ 2009; 35(1):147–54.
39. Chablani SV, Sabra MM. Thyroid cancer and telemedicine during the COVID-19 pandemic. J Endocr Soc 2021;5(6):bvab059.

40. Zhai YK, Zhu WJ, Cai YL, et al. Clinical- and cost-effectiveness of telemedicine in type 2 diabetes mellitus: a systematic review and meta-analysis. Medicine (Baltimore) 2014;93(28):e312.

41. Garg SK, Rodbard D, Hirsch IB, et al. Managing new-onset type 1 diabetes during the COVID-19 pandemic: challenges and opportunities. Diabetes Technol Ther 2020;22(6):431–9.

42. Wang Y, Xue H, Huang Y, et al. A systematic review of application and effectiveness of mhealth interventions for obesity and diabetes treatment and self-management. Adv Nutr 2017;8(3):449–62.

43. Ashrafzadeh S, Hamdy O. Patient-driven diabetes care of the future in the technology era. Cell Metab 2019;29(3):564–75.

44. Miyamoto S, Henderson S, Fazio S, et al. Empowering diabetes self-management through technology and nurse health coaching. Diabetes Educ 2019;45(6):586–95.

45. Lee PA, Greenfield G, Pappas Y. The impact of telehealth remote patient monitoring on glycemic control in type 2 diabetes: a systematic review and meta-analysis of systematic reviews of randomised controlled trials. BMC Health Serv Res 2018;18(1):495.

46. Peters AL, Garg SK. The silver lining to COVID-19: avoiding diabetic ketoacidosis admissions with telehealth. Diabetes Technol Ther 2020;22(6):449–53.

47. Lisco G, De Tullio A, Jirillo E, et al. Thyroid and COVID-19: a review on pathophysiological, clinical and organizational aspects. J Endocrinol Invest 2021; 44(9):1801–14.

48. Siegel CA. Transforming gastroenterology care with telemedicine. Gastroenterology 2017;152(5):958–63.

49. Tang Z, Dubois S, Soon C, et al. A model for the pandemic and beyond: telemedicine for all outpatient gastroenterology referrals reduces unnecessary clinic visits. J Telemed Telecare 2020;20. 1357633X20957224.

50. de Jong MJ, van der Meulen-de Jong AE, Romberg-Camps MJ, et al. Telemedicine for management of inflammatory bowel disease (myIBDcoach): a pragmatic, multicentre, randomised controlled trial. Lancet 2017;390(10098): 959–68.

51. Serper M, Nunes F, Ahmad N, et al. Positive early patient and clinician experience with telemedicine in an academic gastroenterology practice during the COVID-19 pandemic. Gastroenterology 2020;159(4):1589–91, e4.

52. Bensted K, Kim C, Freiman J, et al. Gastroenterology hospital outpatients report high rates of satisfaction with a Telehealth model of care. J Gastroenterol Hepatol 2022;37(1):63–8.

53. Keihanian T, Sharma P, Goyal J, et al. Telehealth utilization in gastroenterology clinics amid the COVID-19 pandemic: impact on clinical practice and gastroenterology training. Gastroenterology 2020;159(4):1598–601.

54. Parmar P, Mackie D, Varghese S, et al. Use of telemedicine technologies in the management of infectious diseases: a review. Clin Infect Dis 2015;60(7): 1084–94.

55. Frank AP, Wandell MG, Headings MD, et al. Anonymous HIV testing using home collection and telemedicine counseling. a multicenter evaluation. Arch Intern Med 1997;157(3):309–14.

56. Touger R, Wood BR. A review of telehealth innovations for HIV pre-exposure prophylaxis (PrEP). Curr Hiv/Aids Rep 2019;16(1):113–9.

57. Smith E, Badowski ME. Telemedicine for HIV care: current status and future prospects. HIV AIDS Auckl 2021;13:651–6.

58. Spinelli MA, Hickey MD, Glidden DV, et al. Viral suppression rates in a safety-net HIV clinic in San Francisco destabilized during COVID-19. AIDS 2020;34(15): 2328–31.

59. Ohl ME, Richardson K, Rodriguez-Barradas MC, et al. Impact of availability of telehealth programs on documented hiv viral suppression: a cluster-randomized program evaluation in the veterans health administration. Open Forum Infect Dis 2019;6(6):ofz206.

60. Dandachi D, Lee C, Morgan RO, et al. Integration of telehealth services in the healthcare system: with emphasis on the experience of patients living with HIV. J Investig Med 2019;67(5):815–20.

61. Tahan V, Almashhrawi A, Mutrux R, et al. Show Me ECHO-Hepatitis C: a telemedicine mentoring program for patients with hepatitis C in underserved and rural areas in Missouri as a model in developing countries. Turk J Gastroenterol 2015;26(6):447–9.

62. Lai S, Farnham A, Ruktanonchai NW, et al. Measuring mobility, disease connectivity and individual risk: a review of using mobile phone data and mHealth for travel medicine. J Travel Med 2019;26(3):taz019.

63. Burnham JP, Fritz SA, Yaeger LH, et al. Telemedicine infectious diseases consultations and clinical outcomes: a systematic review. Open Forum Infect Dis 2019; 6(12):ofz517.

64. Wechsler LR, Tsao JW, Levine SR, et al, American Academy of Neurology Telemedicine Work Group. Teleneurology applications: report of the telemedicine work group of the American academy of neurology. Neurology 2013;80(7): 670–6.

65. Patel UK, Malik P, DeMasi M, et al. Multidisciplinary approach and outcomes of tele-neurology: a review. Cureus 2019;11(4):e4410.

66. Zhai YK, Zhu WJ, Hou HL, et al. Efficacy of telemedicine for thrombolytic therapy in acute ischemic stroke: a meta-analysis. J Telemed Telecare 2015;21(3): 123–30.

67. Hatcher-Martin JM, Adams JL, Anderson ER, et al. Telemedicine in neurology: telemedicine work group of the american academy of neurology update. Neurology 2020;94(1):30–8.

68. Chirra M, Marsili L, Wattley L, et al. Telemedicine in neurological disorders: opportunities and challenges. Telemed J E-health Off J Am Telemed Assoc 2019; 25(7):541–50.

69. Domingues RB, Mantese CE, Aquino E da S, et al. Telemedicine in neurology: current evidence. Arq Neuropsiquiatr 2020;78(12):818–26.

70. Lavin B, Dormond C, Scantlebury MH, et al. Bridging the healthcare gap: building the case for epilepsy virtual clinics in the current healthcare environment. Epilepsy Behav 2020;111:107262.

71. Noutsios CD, Boisvert-Plante V, Perez J, et al. Telemedicine applications for the evaluation of patients with non-acute headache: a narrative review. J Pain Res 2021;14:1533–42.

72. Wechsler LR. Advantages and limitations of teleneurology. JAMA Neurol 2015; 72(3):349–54.

73. Rametta SC, Fridinger SE, Gonzalez AK, et al. Analyzing 2,589 child neurology telehealth encounters necessitated by the COVID-19 pandemic. Neurology 2020;95(9):e1257–66.

74. Olszewski C, Thomson S, Strauss L, et al. Patient experiences with ambulatory telehealth in neurology: results of a mixed-methods study. Neurol Clin Pract 2021;11(6):484–96.

75. Caffery LJ, Taylor M, Gole G, et al. Models of care in tele-ophthalmology: a scoping review. J Telemed Telecare 2019;25(2):106–22.
76. Parikh D, Armstrong G, Liou V, et al. Advances in Telemedicine in ophthalmology. Semin Ophthalmol 2020;35(4):210–5.
77. Ramakrishnan MS, Gilbert AL. Telemedicine in neuro-ophthalmology. Curr Opin Ophthalmol 2021;32(6):499–503.
78. Perez J, Niburski K, Stoopler M, et al. Telehealth and chronic pain management from rapid adaptation to long-term implementation in pain medicine: a narrative review. Pain Rep 2021;6(1):e912.
79. Flynn DM, Eaton LH, McQuinn H, et al. TelePain: primary care chronic pain management through weekly didactic and case-based telementoring. Contemp Clin Trials Commun 2017;8:162–6.
80. Liddy C, Smyth C, Poulin PA, et al. Supporting better access to chronic pain specialists: the champlain BASE™ eConsult service. J Am Board Fam Med 2017;30(6):766–74.
81. Poulin PA, Romanow HC, Cheng J, et al. Offering eConsult to family physicians with patients on a pain clinic wait list: an outreach exercise. J Healthc Qual 2018; 40(5):e71–6.
82. Alter BJ, Navlani R, Abdullah L, et al. The use of telemedicine to support interventional pain care: case series and commentary. Pain Med 2021;22(12): 2802–5.
83. Deer TR, Esposito MF, Cornidez EG, et al. Teleprogramming service provides safe and remote stimulation options for patients with DRG-S and SCS implants. J Pain Res 2021;14:3259–65.
84. Silva LB, Pereira DN, Chagas VS, et al. Orthopedic asynchronous teleconsultation for primary care patients by a large-scale telemedicine service in Minas Gerais, Brazil. Telemed J E-Health 2021;3.
85. Theodore BR, Whittington J, Towle C, et al. Transaction cost analysis of in-clinic versus telehealth consultations for chronic pain: preliminary evidence for rapid and affordable access to interdisciplinary collaborative consultation. Pain Med Malden Mass 2015;16(6):1045–56.
86. Finucane AM, O'Donnell H, Lugton J, et al. Digital health interventions in palliative care: a systematic meta-review. NPJ Digit Med 2021;4(1):64.
87. Allen Watts K, Malone E, Dionne-Odom JN, et al. Can you hear me now?: improving palliative care access through telehealth. Res Nurs Health 2021; 44(1):226–37.
88. Kidd L, Cayless S, Johnston B, et al. Telehealth in palliative care in the UK: a review of the evidence. J Telemed Telecare 2010;16(7):394–402.
89. Oliver DP, Demiris G, Wittenberg-Lyles E, et al. A systematic review of the evidence base for telehospice. Telemed J E-health Off J Am Telemed Assoc 2012;18(1):38–47.
90. Cameron P, Munyan K. Systematic review of telehospice telemedicine and e-health. Telemed J E-health Off J Am Telemed Assoc 2021;27(11):1203–14.
91. Leochico CFD, Mojica JAP, Rey-Matias RR, et al. Role of telerehabilitation in the rehabilitation medicine training program of a COVID-19 referral center in a developing country. Am J Phys Med Rehabil 2021;100(6):526–32.
92. Webster J, Young P, Kiecker J. Telerehabilitation for amputee care. Phys Med Rehabil Clin N Am 2021;32(2):253–62.
93. Subbarao BS, Stokke J, Martin SJ. Telerehabilitation in acquired brain injury. Phys Med Rehabil Clin N Am 2021;32(2):223–38.

94. Havran MA, Bidelspach DE. Virtual physical therapy and telerehabilitation. Phys Med Rehabil Clin N Am 2021;32(2):419–28.

95. Verduzco-Gutierrez M, Lara AM, Annaswamy TM. When disparities and disabilities collide: inequities during the COVID-19 pandemic. PM R 2021;13(4):412–4.

96. Cramer SC, Dodakian L, Le V, et al, National Institutes of Health StrokeNet Telerehab Investigators. Efficacy of home-based telerehabilitation vs in-clinic therapy for adults after stroke: a randomized clinical trial. JAMA Neurol 2019; 76(9):1079–87.

97. Spivak S, Spivak A, Cullen B, et al. Telepsychiatry use in U.S. mental health facilities, 2010-2017. Psychiatr Serv 2020;71(2):121–7.

98. Zachrison KS, Boggs KM, Hayden E, et al. A national survey of telemedicine use by US emergency departments. J Telemed Telecare 2020;26(5):278–84.

99. Fox KC, Connor P, McCullers E, et al. Effect of a behavioural health and specialty care telemedicine programme on goal attainment for youths in juvenile detention. J Telemed Telecare 2008;14(5):227–30.

100. Bashshur RL, Shannon GW, Bashshur N, et al. The empirical evidence for telemedicine interventions in mental disorders. Telemed J E-health Off J Am Telemed Assoc 2016;22(2):87–113.

101. Chen JA, Chung WJ, Young SK, et al. COVID-19 and telepsychiatry: early outpatient experiences and implications for the future. Gen Hosp Psychiatry 2020;66: 89–95.

102. Sasangohar F, Bradshaw MR, Carlson MM, et al. Adapting an outpatient psychiatric clinic to telehealth during the COVID-19 pandemic: a practice perspective. J Med Internet Res 2020;22(10):e22523.

103. Dubin JM, Wyant WA, Balaji NC, et al. Telemedicine usage among urologists during the COVID-19 pandemic: cross-sectional study. J Med Internet Res 2020;22(11):e21875.

104. Nourian A, Smith N, Kleinman L, et al. A 5-year single-institution experience integrating telehealth into urologic care delivery. Telemed E-Health 2021;27(9): 997–1002.

105. Castaneda P, Ellimoottil C. Current use of telehealth in urology: a review. World J Urol 2020;38(10):2377–84.

106. Chao GF, Li KY, Zhu Z, et al. Use of telehealth by surgical specialties during the COVID-19 pandemic. JAMA Surg 2021;156(7):620–6.

107. Gan Z, Lee SY, Weiss DA, et al. Single institution experience with telemedicine for pediatric urology outpatient visits: Adapting to COVID-19 restrictions, patient satisfaction, and future utilization. J Pediatr Urol 2021;17(4):480.e1–7.

108. Chrapah S, Becevic M, Washington KT, et al. Patient and provider satisfaction with pediatric urology telemedicine clinic. J Patient Exp 2021;8. 2374373520975734.

109. Khorsandi N, Gros B, Chiu YW, et al. Telemedicine provides enhanced care for low-acuity pediatric urology patients. Telehealth Med Today 2020;5(3).

110. Canon S, Shera A, Patel A, et al. A pilot study of telemedicine for post-operative urological care in children. J Telemed Telecare 2014;20(8):427–30.

111. Viers BR, Lightner DJ, Rivera ME, et al. Efficiency, satisfaction, and costs for remote video visits following radical prostatectomy: a randomized controlled trial. Eur Urol 2015;68(4):729–35.

112. Park ES, Boedeker BH, Hemstreet JL, et al. The initiation of a preoperative and postoperative telemedicine urology clinic. Stud Health Technol Inform 2011;163: 425–7.

113. Kaczmarek BF, Trinh QD, Menon M, et al. Tablet Telerounding. Urol 2012;80(6): 1383–8.
114. Chu S, Boxer R, Madison P, et al. Veterans affairs telemedicine: bringing urologic care to remote clinics. Urology 2015;86(2):255–60.
115. Medicare and telehealth: coverage and use during the COVID-19 pandemic and options for the future. KFF. 2021. Available at: https://www.kff.org/medicare/issue-brief/medicare-and-telehealth-coverage-and-use-during-the-covid-19-pandemic-and-options-for-the-future/. Accessed December 11, 2021.
116. Patel SY, Mehrotra A, Huskamp HA, et al. Variation in telemedicine use and outpatient care during the COVID-19 pandemic in the United States. Health Aff (Millwood) 2021;40(2):349–58.
117. Alkureishi MA, Choo ZY, Rahman A, et al. Digitally disconnected: qualitative study of patient perspectives on the digital divide and potential solutions. JMIR Hum Factors 2021;8(4):e33364.
118. Javier-DesLoges J, Meagher M, Soliman S, et al. Disparities in telemedicine utilization for urology patients during the COVID-19 pandemic. Urology 2021;4295: 01193–6. Published online December 31.
119. Liu X, Goldenthal S, Li M, et al. Comparison of telemedicine versus in-person visits on impact of downstream utilization of care. Telemed J E-health Off J Am Telemed Assoc 2021;27(10):1099–104.
120. Calendar year (CY) 2022 medicare physician fee schedule final rule | CMS. 2021. Available at: https://www.cms.gov/newsroom/fact-sheets/calendar-year-cy-2022-medicare-physician-fee-schedule-final-rule. Accessed December 11.

Telehealth and Medical Education

Aleksandr Belakovskiy, MD*, Elizabeth K. Jones, MD

KEYWORDS

- Telehealth • Telemedicine • Medical education • Medical students • Residents
- Resident education

KEY POINTS

- Ensure learners are fully equipped to engage in telehealth visits.
- Medical educators should be prepared to give meaningful feedback specific to telehealth.
- Both learners and medical educators should be aware of the benefits and limitations of telehealth visits.

INTRODUCTION

Telehealth in outpatient primary care has been present for over a decade but saw a dramatic expansion during the COVID-19 pandemic.[1] For resident physicians in primary care, virtual visits have expanded the ability to deliver patient care. This was initially done out of necessity, particularly in March through June of 2020, and to limit exposure to COVID-19. However, it also removed barriers to patient care including lack of transportation and inadequate time for in-person visits. As telehealth expanded across all specialties in medicine, it became an important component to integrate into medical education. Suddenly, there was a need for learners to be proficient in a new patient care paradigm. The growth of telehealth in primary care has led to the need for curricular change at the undergraduate and graduate levels.

HISTORY

According to a 2016 study, there was a limited amount of literature on the topic of telehealth education. Edirippulige and Armfield explained that there were only 9 studies with substantial review of education and training in telemedicine. Of those 9 studies, only 2 studies originated from the United States.[2] One of the US articles evaluated the impact of telemedicine at the University of Wisconsin nursing program.[3] This study focused on faculty education surrounding telehealth and then incorporation of

University of Michigan Medical School, 300 North Ingalls Street, NI4C06, Ann Arbor, MI 48109, USA
* Corresponding author. Department of Family Medicine, 300 North Ingalls Street, NI4C06, Ann Arbor, MI 48109-5435.
E-mail address: abelakov@med.umich.edu

Prim Care Clin Office Pract 49 (2022) 575–583
https://doi.org/10.1016/j.pop.2022.04.003

telehealth into the nursing curriculum. Faculty were surveyed before and after the faculty development intervention and showed improved comfort with telehealth. The other article focused on the evaluation of an online curriculum for Veteran Affairs (VA) staff without clear indication of whether physicians were included in this study.[4] Participants felt that the VA online curriculum overall improved telehealth skills with the most frequently cited areas of improvement being telehealth operations (32%), roles and duties (22%), marketing strategies (18%), program implementation (17%), and patient selection methodologies (13%). The limited studies on education in telehealth illustrate the sparsity of curricula prior to the COVID-19 pandemic, especially among US-based learners, and suggest the imminent need for guidance.

As of 2021, there has been significant acceleration in the role of telehealth curricula. The Society of Teachers of Family Medicine (STFM) developed an online curriculum to reflect the increasing role of telemedicine, STFM Telemedicine Curriculum. This online curriculum focuses on the current role of telehealth, the logistics of performing telehealth, and the role of health equity in virtual care.[5] The STFM curriculum was developed for all learners including medical students, residents, faculty, and community preceptors. Separately, a single-center study conducted during the pandemic highlighted the implementation of a telemedicine curriculum for internal medicine residents.[6] The aim of the study was to evaluate a novel telehealth curriculum for internal medicine residents in a primary care setting. Most residents said that a formal telemedicine curriculum was relevant to patient care and would improve their ability to deliver care in future encounters.

HEALTH EQUITY

Telehealth allows for increased access to health care by limiting barriers such as geographic distance, transportation, need for time off work, and need for childcare. However, it disproportionately benefits those with greater financial resources and technology literacy. As of April 2021, there were still significantly lower rates of Internet use among individuals aged 65 years or older and individuals with annual income less than $30,000.[7] A study conducted in a single academic primary care department examined the impact of initiating telemedicine during the COVID-19 pandemic. While comparing a 2-week period before implementation of video and telephone visits with a 2 period after beginning telehealth visits, video visits increased from 3% to 80%, and telephone visits increased from 0% to 16%. However, there was a reduction in visits (type of visit was not specified) for those 65 and older (41% to 35%, $P=.002$), non-English language preference (14% to 7%, $P<.001$), and Medicaid and Medicare users (43% to 22%, $P<.001$.)[8] These studies illustrate the disparities in access to telehealth based on social determinants of health.

From an educational perspective, telehealth is another area of health care where social determinants of health and equity must be taught explicitly. A 2006 article on social justice in medical education stated "it becomes absurd to teach social justice as a subject matter, a skill set or knowledge base; rather, by teaching all relevant subjects, including social issues, in a new way, social justice becomes an integral part of the process of education itself."[9] When teaching and incorporating telemedicine in clinical practice, it is important for learners of all levels to be mindful of the limitations and utility of this method of care.

DISCUSSION

Considering the importance of telehealth education and experience for medical learners, along with the relative dearth of recommendations about how to provide such an experience for learners in primary care, the authors propose a novel, yet standardized, approach to telehealth encounters with a learner. The steps include preparation, observation, assessment, and feedback. These steps have significant overlap with in-person clinical teaching, and a medical educator's experience in this realm should be leveraged for optimal teaching in telehealth. Each step is outlined in detail, along with an overview of the authors' recommended approach in **Fig. 1**.

Preparation

An important first step before a virtual visit is to prepare the learner for the session. Having shared expectations among teacher and learner regarding the number of patients to be seen, how to reach each other for questions, and the type(s) of observation expected for each visit will allow for a smooth transition to the virtual day of health care. It is important to have accessible ways to reach each other and for the learner to be able to ask questions during the patient care session if the educator and learner are not physically together.[10] Specifically for medical students, it is important to set the expectation that they do not need to see every patient. In fact, 3 to 4 patients in a half-day session generally allows for variety in patients seen while also leaving time for reading and feedback.[5] It is also important to set expectations before the session regarding any documentation the learner is required to submit and for how many patients. Lastly, it is recommended to engage learners to set learning goals for themselves, as this will allow for targeted and tailored teaching and feedback.

Observation

Similar to in-person observation of medical students and resident physicians during a clinical encounter, there are several ways to observe learner/patient interactions during a telehealth encounter.[5] Before the clinical session, there should be a shared expectation related to the type of observation for each encounter. Common options include being present for the entire visit, joining the visit after the history and virtual physical examination are completed but before assessment and plan, or an asynchronous discussion of the patient case (**Table 1**).

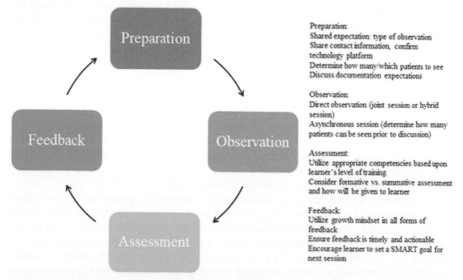

Fig. 1. Cycle of teaching in the telehealth encounter.

Table 1
Options for Observation

Format	Example
Joint session	Student/resident calls patient or joins video visit at same time as preceptor. The supervising physician is able to directly observe the entire encounter in real time. This allows for in depth feedback to the learner and ability for the preceptor to engage in the plan for the patient at the time of visit.
Hybrid session	Student/resident calls a patient or joins a video visit and conducts history and physical examination. Learner contacts the preceptor via a predetermined method to discuss the case. It is important if using the video visit platform to precept the case without the patient present to only discuss that patient's case because of HIPAA (Health Insurance Portability and Accountability Act of 1996) concerns. Learner and preceptor join visit together to discuss plan with patient. Preceptor is able to directly observe the learner's interaction with patients related to communication and patient education as the plan is discussed.
Asynchronous session	Resident completes the entire visit independently and discusses the case afterward with the preceptor. This is not recommended for medical student learners. There should be shared understanding before the visit about how quickly a resident should contact the preceptor after each case, and there should be a reliable way to reach the preceptor during visit for any questions or urgent concerns.

A major strength of using telehealth for direct observation of medical learners is the ability for the physician to turn off a camera or mute one's phone in order to unobtrusively monitor the encounter, which enables specific and high-quality feedback of interview skills.[11] The mode of the telehealth encounter may impact observation abilities. For example, during a video encounter, the physician observer is able to view facial expressions, mannerisms, and professional backgrounds, while this is not possible during phone encounters.

Many facets of observation will be similar to direct observation in person, including monitoring the content and efficiency of history taking and ability to appropriately communicate plans and deliver patient education. In a telehealth visit, the teaching physician should make particular note of the learner's webside manner, such as eye contact, talking speed, tone, body language, and nonverbal cues.[5] The teaching physician should also note if the learner conducts an appropriate physical examination for the virtual environment, when relevant, if at all.

Assessment

The assessment of learners' use of telehealth should be targeted to their level of training. The Association of American Medical Colleges (AAMC) has developed a helpful guide in this domain as published in Telehealth Competencies Across the Learning Continuum,[12] based on expert consensus regarding the most important telehealth skills required for health care professionals.[13] These competencies are organized into 6 domains and over 3 tiers of development, detailed in **Table 2**.

Robust literature does not yet exist regarding options for application of evaluation tools in telehealth. One internal medicine residency program created a mini-clinical evaluation exercise (mini-CEX) for telemedicine.[6] These evaluations were sent to faculty before virtual visits and asked for actionable feedback on individual virtual encounters via 7 questions based up the 6 ACGME core competencies of patient care, medical knowledge, practice-based learning and improvement, inter-personal and communication skills, professionalism and systems-based practice.[14]

Table 2 Association of American Medical Colleges telehealth competencies	
Domains	Patient safety and appropriate use of telehealth Access and equity in telehealth Communication via telehealth Data collection and assessment via telehealth Ethical practices and legal requirements for telehealth
Tiers of developmental stages	Entry to residency or recent medical school graduate Entry to practice or recent residency graduate Experienced faculty physician or 3 to 5 years post-residency

Data from Association of American Medical Colleges (AAMC). Telehealth Competencies Across the Learning Continuum. AAMC New and Emerging Areas in Medicine Series. Washington, DC: AAMC; 2021.

Until more specific tools are created for evaluation in telehealth, using ACGME core competencies and the learning objectives outlined in the STFM Telemedicine Curriculum may allow for educator organization of learner assessment in this area.

Feedback

The final crucial step in telehealth education is to provide feedback to the learner that is useful and actionable. Similar to in-person precepting, there are multiple ways in which to provide this feedback. First, if at all possible, it is important for this feedback to be timely following the interaction. Providing feedback at the end of the session is optimal in order to recall important details of the learner's performance. Starting a brief feedback session by asking the learner what he or she thought went well and what he or she thought could be improved is recommended. Feedback can then be tailored based on the learner's goals set during the preparation stage. There are many resources for providing useful feedback; making it specific, actionable, and useful is of paramount importance. The One-Minute Preceptor model is 1 such model allowing for rapid feedback during a clinical session, by following the 5 microskills of: getting a commitment, probing for supporting evidence, teaching general rules, reinforcing what was done right, and correcting mistakes.[15] The ARCH model is another tool that may be used with the steps of allowing for self-assessment; reinforcing correct behavior, knowledge, and/or attitudes; correcting incorrect behavior and/or knowledge, and helping the learner with an improvement plan.[16]

Overall, the authors recommend approaching feedback with a growth-mindset frame of reference. This involves moving from a fixed mindset of success as something innate and unchangeable to a growth mindset that success results from hard work, learning, and training and that there is much to be learned from failure. A growth mindset pushes learners to consider constructive feedback and incorporate it into ongoing reflective practice for improvement.[17] From this perspective, feedback is grounded in specific observations based on learner goals in order to continuously improve.[18] Keeping feedback brief and limited to 1 or 2 areas allows for manageable amounts of information is most useful for learners in medical training. Offering specific feedback about the learner's webside manner and utilization of the technology for the visit is of particular importance during telehealth visits. At the conclusion of feedback, asking the learner to set an SMART goal (specific, measurable, attainable, realistic, and time bound) for the next session will allow for continuous improvement.[19]

In summary, many of the central tenets of in-person clinical education are applicable to telehealth medical education. This is a rapidly evolving field with a lack of consistent guidelines for recommendations regarding approaches to telehealth education. Therefore, the authors have created a standardized approach, and **Fig. 1** summarizes our proposed cycle for optimal teaching of the telehealth encounter.

CASE STUDIES
Case Study 1 Resident Care of Hypertension via Virtual Visit

Presentation
A 45-year-old man presents for a follow-up for poorly controlled hypertension. His past medical history is significant for obstructive sleep apnea, primary hypertension, and hyperlipidemia. He was previously evaluated in the clinic 2 weeks prior, at which time his blood pressure was 150/90. He has a blood pressure cuff at home that has been validated for accuracy in the clinic. He is currently taking amlodipine 10 mg once daily, follows the Dietary Approaches to Stop Hypertension (DASH) diet, and uses his continuous positive airway pressure (CPAP) nightly for 8 hours every night. Today, he reports he has been checking his blood pressure every day twice daily and following instructions for proper blood pressure measuring. His blood pressure has averaged 150/85 over the last 2 weeks.

Clinical question
What would be the next steps in managing this patient's blood pressure via telehealth?

Discussion
This case illustrates several points that are germane to residents providing care through telemedicine. Chronic diseases like hypertension are well suited for virtual care, as they often do not involve seeking new physical examination findings or extensive evaluation. The caveat for hypertension is that patients will need to have a reliable way to check their own blood pressure to guide management. If the patient has a reliable way to check and report his or her hypertension, then virtual care can remove barriers to care such as transportation, arranging childcare, and missing time for work. However, it is crucial to be mindful that this assumes a patient can acquire a blood pressure cuff, accurately measure, and record blood pressures. There are numerous factors that may limit a patient's ability to check their own blood pressure including but not limited to, manual dexterity, sufficient vision, an appropriately calibrated blood pressure cuff, and financial resources. It is important for residents to be mindful of these factors as they develop a plan for monitoring a patient with hypertension.

Furthermore, if one were to add a new agent such as a thiazide diuretic or angiotensin converting enzyme (ACE) inhibitor, it is common practice to obtain a basic metabolic panel to establish baseline renal function and to evaluate for electrolyte abnormalities or an acute kidney injury. As telehealth expands the ability to care for patients outside of our direct communities, it is prudent to think of how patients can complete follow-up care such as obtaining laboratory studies in a timely fashion. As the prescribing physician, house officers must be mindful of how patients can follow through with plans if they are not located near their primary care office.

Although there are several aspects of this case that can be highlighted, a key takeaway is the importance of house officers to understand the barriers to carrying out a care plan. This can be made simpler or more difficult when conducting a telehealth visit. As learners are trained on providing care in the virtual space, it is important to be mindful of the differences in providing care through a virtual platform.

Case Study 2: Teaching Anxiety Management via Telehealth

Case presentation

A 60-year-old woman has a video visit scheduled with her primary care physician (you) to discuss management of ongoing anxiety symptoms. She was diagnosed with generalized anxiety disorder 5 years ago, which was previously well managed with an ongoing relationship with a therapist, meditation, and hydroxyzine taken on an as needed basis. Over the last 4 months, she has noticed increasing anxiety, daily feelings of worry that have led to difficulty falling asleep, decreased sleep time, and fatigue during the day. You have a family medicine clerkship medical student working with you who will participate in this virtual visit.

Clinical questions

What are the next steps in evaluation and management of anxiety in this patient? How can you best observe and teach the medical student working with you for virtual care?

Discussion

Preparation for this session would include having a shared expectation with the student regarding type of contact that will occur between the two of you as you are not in the same physical location and plan for type of observation. Before the virtual visit, the student should have your preferred contact information (in this case, you prefer texting), understanding that you will use the electronic health records (EHR)'s Zoom (or other similar virtual platform) function to conduct the visit and that you will provide feedback after the visit within the Zoom visit. You will let the student know ahead of time that he or she will be gathering the history and that it will be a hybrid session in which he or she will gather the history, then present the case to you including a plan, followed by both of you returning to the room for direct observation of the student discussing the plan with Ms. Smith. You can then assess the student's presentation skills and medical knowledge as you would in person. The virtual environment allows for you to observe the student's webside manner and ability to ask pertinent questions, noting if he or she remarks upon or asks about the patient's mental status and home environment as seen on the video. You are then able to give feedback directly after the session, teaching about pearls of anxiety management, use of standardized forms in psychiatric care (eg, Patient Health Questionnaire [PHQ]-9 and General Anxiety Disorder [GAD]-7 forms). For example, if the student did not consider use of these forms, then this could be part of his or her SMART goal for future sessions related to anxiety management. Lastly, feedback would include encouraging the student to present a care plan and feedback about the accuracy and feasibility of this plan. Use of the One-Minute Preceptor model of feedback would be a possible strategy in this case.[17]

Case Study 3: Teaching the Importance of Triage in Telehealth

Case presentation

A 25-year-old woman is scheduled for an urgent video visit with you for 1 day of lower left abdominal pain.

Clinical questions

What are the next steps in evaluation and management of abdominal pain in this patient? How do you best prepare, observe, and teach the medical student working with you for virtual care?

Discussion

Although virtual visits expand ability to provide care, they may lead to patients being scheduled who would be better managed via in-person visit because of the need for physical examination or real-time testing. In this case, focusing on use of telehealth as a mode of triage could be an effective educational goal. This would start with adequate preparation for the visit with the medical student. The authors recommend preparing the student for a hybrid form of observation in which the student will ask the patient relevant questions while you observe. Next, having a discussion with the student during preparation stage about red flags that must be asked of the patient to triage next steps. In this case, ensuring the student is aware of issues such as possibility of pregnancy, risk for sexually transmitted infections as cause of pelvic inflammatory disease, expanded gastrointestinal review of systems to evaluate for inflammatory bowel disease and symptoms of bowel obstruction are critical. Following the hybrid observation of the student, assessment and feedback will focus on the student's knowledge of the red flags and history taking skills. Lastly, the authors recommend using similar cases to highlight some of the limitations of telehealth as a modality of care.

CLINICS CARE POINTS

1. Learner Access to Technology: Learners must have access to a telephone and a device capable of video visits. Furthermore, they must have access to a stable, reliable Internet connection to limit disruptions in video telehealth visits if they are not conducting such visits from the ambulatory office practice.

2. Patient Access to Technology: Similarly, this model of health care delivery is predicated on patients having access to video-enabled devices, telephones, stable Internet service, and active telephone lines. Furthermore, patients need to have the technology literacy to use devices.

3. Appropriateness of the Visit: Certain health conditions may lend themselves poorly to telehealth, such as those requiring a detailed physical examination, in-house laboratory assessment, or testing evaluation via electrocardiogram.

4. Interpreter Services: It is important to have access to interpreter services in a telehealth setting and to choose the appropriate form of telehealth (eg, video visit for American Sign Language interpretation).

5. Professionalism: Learners should be mindful of their attire when engaging patients in telehealth visits. Furthermore, they should be mindful of their backgrounds, including distractions such as pictures and paintings.

6. Billing: As billing parameters evolve and change, it is important to be mindful of the implications on virtual visits. This includes how virtual visits (telephone vs video) are billed and supervision of residents and fellows.

DISCLOSURE

The authors have no relevant disclosures.

REFERENCES

1. Hong YR, Lawrence J, Williams D Jr, et al. Population-level interest and telehealth capacity of US hospitals in response to COVID-19: cross-sectional analysis of google search and national hospital survey data. JMIR Public Health Surveill 2020;6(2):e18961.

2. Edirippulige S, Armfield NR. Education and training to support the use of clinical telehealth: a review of the literature. J Telemed Telecare 2017;23(2):273–82.
3. Gallagher-Lepak S, Scheibel P, Gibson C. Integrating telehealth in nursing curricula: can you hear me now. Online J Nurs Info 2009;13:1–16.
4. Kobb RF, Lane RJ, Stallings D. E-learning and telehealth: measuring your success. Telemed J E Health 2008;14(6):576–9.
5. Lin S., Bajra R., Banning R., et al., S. STFM telemedicine curriculum. Retrieved from STFM.org. Available at: https://www.stfm.org/teachingresources/curriculum/telemedicine/telemedicinecurriculum/#24129, 2021. Accessed October 18, 2021.
6. Savage DJ, Gutierrez O, Montané BE, et al. Implementing a telemedicine curriculum for internal medicine residents during a pandemic: the Cleveland Clinic experience. Postgrad Med J 2021. https://doi.org/10.1136/postgradmedj-2020-139228. Epub ahead of print.
7. Pew Research Center. Internet/broadband fact sheet [Internet] Pew Res Cent Internet Technol. 2019. Available at: https://www.pewresearch.org/internet/fact-sheet/internet-broadband/. Accessed October 18, 2021.
8. Nouri SS, Khoong EC, Lyles CR, et al. Addressing equity in telemedicine for chronic disease management during the COVID-19 pandemic. NEJM Catal [Internet; 2020. p. 1–13.
9. DasGupta S, Fornari A, Geer K, et al. Medical education for social justice: Paulo Freire revisited. J Med Humanit 2006;27:245–51.
10. Wamsley M, Cornejo L, Kryzhanovskaya I, et al. Best practices for integrating medical students into telehealth visits. JMIR Med Educ 2021;7(2):e27877.
11. Stumbar S, Lee A, Erlich D, et al. STFM education columns. Overcoming challenges in webside teaching: results of an SWOT analysis at the 2021 STFM conference on medical student education. Available at: https://stfm.org/publicationsresearch/publications/educationcolumns/2021/november/. Accessed on December 1, 2021.
12. AAMC. Telehealth Competencies Across the Learning Continuum. AAMC New and Emerging Areas in Medicine Series. Washington (DC): AAMC; 2021.
13. Galpin K, Sikka N, King SL, et al, AAMC Telehealth Advisory Committee. Expert consensus: telehealth skills for health care professionals. Telemed J E Health 2021;27(7):820–4.
14. Swing SR. The ACGME outcome project: retrospective and prospective. Med Teach 2007;29(7):648–54.
15. Neher J, Gordon K, Meyer B, et al. A five-step microskills model of clinical teaching. J Am Board Fam Pract 1992;5:419–24.
16. Baker S, Turner G, Bush S. STFM education columns. ARCH: a guidance model for providing effective feedback to learners. Available at: https://www.stfm.org/publicationsresearch/publications/educationcolumns/2015/november/. Accessed on January 18, 2022.
17. Dweck CS. Mindset: the new psychology of success. New York: Random House; 2006.
18. Ramani S, Könings KD, Ginsburg S, et al. Twelve tips to promote a feedback culture with a growth mind-set: swinging the feedback pendulum from recipes to relationships. Med Teach 2019;41(6):625–31.
19. Conzemius A, O'Neill J. The power of SMART goals: using goals to improve student learning. Solution Tree Press; 2009.

Use of Telehealth in Pediatrics

Andrea B. Buchi, MD[a],*, Debra M. Langlois, MD[b], Rebecca Northway, MD[b,c]

KEYWORDS

- Telehealth • Telemedicine • Pediatric • COVID-19

KEY POINTS

- Changes in laws related to the billing of telehealth encounters are ongoing and many are temporary under the Public Health Emergency.
- Telehealth can be quite useful in caring for the Pediatric population with a variety of chronic and acute conditions, including mental and behavioral health.
- Telehealth promotes the medical home and expands access to pediatric specialists.
- Incorporating learners into telehealth can have challenges but is an important learning opportunity and an essential skill they must learn before independent practice.

INTRODUCTION

Telehealth is an important avenue to provide care for our pediatric patients. It is likely that most readers received little to no training in telehealth during their instructional training outside of after-hours telephone calls from patients and their families. However, telehealth now encompasses a wide variety of interactions between patients and providers as well as between primary care and specialists (**Table 1**).

The COVID-19 pandemic has required overnight adaptation to a wide variety of telehealth modalities, most notably video visits. Early 2020 saw the closure of many businesses, schools, and even medical clinics in an attempt to stop the spread of COVID-19, which fueled the rapid expansion of telehealth. Telehealth utilization in the United States was at 1% of all visits at the end of February 2020[1] and increased to more than 50% 5 weeks later.[2] Similarly, in week 13 of 2020 telehealth visits increased 154% compared with the same week in 2019.[3] Emergency changes in laws allowed physicians to bill for encounters in ways that were previously more limited. Patients and families have eagerly adapted to this new way of interacting

[a] Department of Pediatrics and Virtual Care, University of Michigan, 400 E. Eisenhower Parkway, Building 2, Suite B, Ann Arbor, MI 48108, USA; [b] Department of Pediatrics, University of Michigan, 1051 North Canton Center Road, Canton, MI 48187, USA; [c] Department of Internal Medicine, Primary Care Sports Medicine, University of Michigan, 1051 North Canton Center Road, Canton, MI 48187, USA
* Corresponding author.
E-mail address: abraunz@med.umich.edu

Prim Care Clin Office Pract 49 (2022) 585–596
https://doi.org/10.1016/j.pop.2022.04.005
0095-4543/22/© 2022 Elsevier Inc. All rights reserved.

Table 1
Types of telehealth encounters, how they relate and differ from each other, and their definitions

	Synchronous	Asynchronous
Patient to provider	Video visit Phone visit	Portal Message E-visit Remote patient monitoring
Provider to provider	Teleconsult	E-consult

Synchronous: A live or real-time interaction between 2 or more parties.

Asynchronous: A written communication between 2 or more parties that may or may not allow for a response. Commonly referred to as "store and forward" in telehealth.

Video visit: Audio and video connection used to conduct a patient encounter.

Phone visit: Audio-only connection used to conduct a patient encounter.

Portal message: A written message or question sent to/from a patient to/from a provider, similar to an e-mail, but within the medical chart.

E-visit: A patient completed a questionnaire that is sent to a provider to provide care for relatively straight-forward illnesses and conditions.

Remote patient monitoring (RPM): A standardized collection of data that is then transmitted using technology to the provider for review(ie: weight, blood pressure, glucometer).

Teleconsult: Audio and or/video connection between 2 or more providers to provide real-time care and advice for a patient.

E-consult: A provider completed a questionnaire that is sent to a specialist for advice on the diagnosis and/or management of a condition that the submitting provider plans to manage.

with their providers, making it very unlikely to ever go away. In fact, further analysis[4] of medical claims records from January 1, 2020 through January 25, 2021 shows elevated levels of telehealth adoption for behavioral health (71.3%) and primary care (23.7%) compared with medical (17.1%) and surgical (5.2%) specialties, making this particularly pertinent to all pediatric providers.

The levels of telehealth adoption have stabilized and as of January 2021, pediatric patients (0–17 yr) and their parents (18–44 yr) lead at 24% and 21%, respectively, compared with 19% of 45 to 65 year olds and 14% of 65+ year olds.[4] This shows that our patients and their families are willing and ready to continue to access care via telehealth. In fact they will demand we offer it or they may seek care elsewhere.[5] This article will explore applications for telehealth related to pediatrics.

DISCUSSION
Telehealth Billing and Insurance Coverage During the COVID-19 Pandemic

For the most part, billing for a telehealth encounter with pediatric patients is the same as for adult patients. One notable difference is that a well-child examination cannot be billed via telehealth[6] which differs from the Medicare annual wellness visit, which does not require a physical examination.[7] Before the COVID-19 pandemic, most telehealth was not covered by insurance and many providers were uncomfortable billing for such services due to complex and confusing rules.

Under the Public Health Emergency (PHE)[8] for COVID-19 as declared by the Secretary of Health and Human Services under section 319 of the Public Health Service Act, the complex rules for telehealth billing were relaxed to allow patients to receive care while limiting exposure to COVID-19. The main difference between the existing policy and the PHE is that patients are allowed to be in their nonrural homes at the time of the telehealth visit.[3,9,10] Reimbursement is complex and changing frequently thus is beyond the scope of this article. The PHE changes are subject to end or change when the PHE expires (last renewed for 90 days on April 16, 2022).[11]

While both new patient visits and return patient visits are eligible to be seen virtually, it is important to consider that a telehealth visit may not be the optimal way to meet a new patient, particularly a newborn.[5,6] Most states require the patient to be in the state whereby the provider is licensed,[10,12] but this can be in their home, car, or another available location. This flexibility is what many patients love about telehealth.

Historically, patients are not accustomed to being billed for advice given over the telephone or via a patient portal message. Answering these requests does take time and effort from providers. As these are a form of telehealth, providers should consider billing these encounters to insurance. As we all adjust to this new coverage, transparency regarding billing is essential to maintaining good relationships between patient and provider.

Considerations for Pediatric Telehealth Encounters

Four important aspects to consider with pediatric telehealth are privacy, participants, obtaining vitals, and consideration of laboratories. In contrast to in-person visits, ensuring privacy during a telehealth encounter may be more challenging. Even if only the patient is visible during the visit, it is possible there are others around. We recommend asking if others are present and, if so, confirming your ability to share confidential information. If additional providers are present, including clinical learners, all attempts should be made to have them visible as well; however, if this is not possible the patient should be informed of their presence and if they leave or reenter the encounter space.[13]

It is generally assumed that a pediatric patient will be present during all in-office encounters. However, with telehealth, it is possible that the parent may not think to include the patient. Training your support staff to remind parents when the child's presence is required can prevent last-minute cancellations and rescheduling of telehealth visits. An advantage to telehealth is that multiple family members can be involved, even from different locations. This can be particularly beneficial when in-office space is limited or family members do not live together.

When a pediatric patient is seen in-person vital signs are measured. Telehealth vitals are limited by remote monitoring technology available and parent's comfort and skill level. For larger patients where weight is measured in pounds only, a home scale can suffice. But for infants, a more precise weight is needed. If an infant scale is not available, a digital cooking scale can be used for smaller babies. If no weight is available and a weight-based medication is being prescribed, make sure to consider the date of the last weight in the chart and how likely it is to still apply based on the child's age. Some smartphones and fitness watches can now check heart rates, blood pressures, and oxygen saturations. Results must be interpreted with caution as there are potentials for user or technological error. Furthermore, an appropriately sized pediatric cuff is not always accessible. If reviewing a BP obtained by a patient, remember to confirm the appropriate cuff size.

Coordination of laboratories is an important consideration in deciding if a patient should be seen in-person or via telehealth. For routine monitoring, it may be beneficial to have patients get laboratories drawn in advance so the results can be discussed during the visit. For chief complaints such as sore throat or UTI whereby laboratories are expected, it may not make sense to start with a virtual visit.[3,14]

Equity and Accessibility

Equitable access to medical care is a universal concern, and telehealth can both lessen and exacerbate barriers to receiving medical care. For patients that struggle to get to our offices due to transportation or physical limitation issues, telehealth may improve access to medical care.[15] It can also extend access to pediatric care and specialists for those living in more rural areas of the country.[16] Certain populations may not have access to, or possession of, a device with a camera and high-speed internet connection.[5,10] Lack of technology and/or lack of technology literacy may create barriers to some patients receiving care virtually.[3]

For children with special health care needs (CSHCN) in particular, telehealth can improve their access to care. CSHCN require frequent visits with their primary care physician (PCP) and various pediatric specialists. Using telehealth can allow families to spend less money on transportation and child care arrangements, and may reduce loss of time at work for parents.[17] In a 2004 study, before experiencing a telehealth encounter, only 50% of families with CSHCN indicated they would be "very likely" to use telehealth in the future, while after they experienced a telehealth encounter, 98% of those families wished to continue to receive the specialty consultations via telehealth.[18]

Remote patient monitoring tools allow more complex care to be conducted virtually. There are commercially available products that allow patients to take audio recordings of their breathing and heart sounds, and video recordings and photos of their skin, throats, and tympanic membranes. While information from these remote patient monitoring devices may improve diagnosis and help with antibiotic stewardship, they may also promote inequity as they can be quite costly.

It is important to continue to use interpreters for non-English speaking patients.[6] Services such as closed captions or live transcription can assist those who are deaf or have difficulty hearing. Literacy levels vary and patients may struggle to understand complex written instructions or navigate the steps needed to prepare for the video visit.

Barriers to Implementing Telehealth in Pediatrics

Before the COVID-19 pandemic, various surveys found that only 12% to 16% of physicians, including pediatricians, were regularly using telehealth as part of their practices. Barriers cited included concern about reimbursement, cost of equipment/ services, and lack of training.[19] While many offices initiated or increased the use of telehealth visits as a result of the pandemic PCPs still expressed frustration with billing and reimbursement.[19]

Additional barriers have been pediatricians' perceived lack of usefulness in their practice and lack of confidence in diagnosis via telehealth.[19] Telehealth visits have been successfully used in various pediatric specialties, but less so formally in general pediatrics, even though many pediatricians have actually been engaging in various forms of telehealth. Pediatricians have traditionally been calling patients or parents while on call or when following up on a nurse triage to evaluate and assess concerns to provide a treatment plan. This is often conducted without the use of a formal examination, but rather via pointed questions and assessment over the phone. With the advent of platforms for video visits, providers can now triage with a visual assessment. This can provide a more reliable and efficient assessment of the patient.

Benefits of Telehealth in Pediatrics

The patient-centered medical home model offers a single "home" for the optimal coordination of all medical care. According to an American Academy of Pediatrics (AAP) policy statement, "Telehealth is a critical infrastructure to efficiently implement the medical home model of care and provide high-value, coordinated, and unfragmented health care."[16] With busy schedules and fears of missing more work or school, many patients and families turn to urgent cares, emergency rooms, and even commercial direct-to-consumer (DTC) video visit encounters for their care, largely due to convenience[5] thus fragmenting their medical home. Telehealth offered through the PCP's office maintains the patient's medical home and continuity of care[15,16] while providing quality, fast care.[15]

Telehealth reduces the time that the patient is missing from school, and time that the parent is missing from work. Miles saved traveling also translates to financial savings for families, as gas for transportation is not needed for telehealth.[18,20] In a study by Johnson and colleagues,[20] families with a telehealth appointment saved an average of 16 miles compared with an in-person primary care visit. In the COVID-19 pandemic, fewer patients being seen in the clinic helps with social distancing and conservation of personal protective equipment. And with visitor restrictions in the COVID-19 pandemic, telehealth allows for the inclusion of additional family members in patient care.

Telehealth also expands pediatric specialty access and access to health extenders. E-consults (see **Table 1**) offered by pediatric specialists can help coordinate care between PCPs and pediatric specialists. One study[21] showed that E-consults conducted with neurology and gastroenterology were able to defer 18% of specialty visits, expedite 21%, and reduce appointment wait times from 48 to 34 days for those patients that needed to be seen directly by the pediatric specialist. For patients who live in areas underserved by pediatric subspecialists, telehealth offers access to pediatric specialty care.

Unexpected benefits have arisen through the use of telehealth in pediatrics. Patients can be observed in their home, and in their natural environment. This can help with developmental observations and identification of psychosocial concerns.[10] A telehealth appointment performed in the patient's home also offers a unique opportunity to perform a home assessment and safety evaluation for pediatric patients.

Limitations and Challenges to Telehealth in Pediatrics

Examinations are limited when a patient is evaluated through telehealth. Telephone visits inherently lack a visual examination, relying on parent description and audible findings from the patient. Video assessment for symptoms involving sensitive areas of the body for pediatric patients requires utmost caution, as there are patient privacy and safety concerns (see Sexual Health section later in discussion). Opportunities for vaccination are missed when a patient is evaluated through telehealth and not in-person. The home environment can be distracting during a telehealth visit. Ensuring adolescent patient confidentiality can be more complicated. Antibiotic stewardship is a concern, if patients are treated empirically for strep throat or a urinary tract infection without appropriate laboratory testing.[14,22] Interpersonal interactions are different during a telehealth visit versus in-person visits. Providers have also experienced inappropriate language and behavior, (ie, parents driving during telehealth visits) which require unique approaches to address.

Common Pediatric Office Visits

The most common visits to the pediatrician's office include well-child examinations, immunization discussion and administration, evaluation for fever and acute illness including common colds and ear infections, and behavioral issues. In-person visits can pose logistical barriers to patients including scheduling conflicts, travel time to appointments, and waiting in a physician's office. Applications of telehealth can be appropriate for many pediatric office visits. Although there are limitations, the use of telehealth within primary care offices could increase access to high-quality pediatric care as well as patient and physician satisfaction, however, further study is needed.

Reassuringly, in a study by McConnochie, et al,[23] except for upper respiratory infections with ear symptoms, there was high agreement in diagnosis between an in-person evaluation and a telehealth evaluation.

Well-Child Care

Well-child examinations are critical to pediatric medicine, providing the foundation for the medical home. The COVID-19 pandemic resulted in a delay of well-child examinations for many children for multiple reasons, including the reduction of in office visits and fear by parents and families to enter the office. The significant decline in well-child visits in 2020 has prompted concern by the AAP because of the resultant delay in vaccinations, anticipatory guidance, and age-appropriate screening and necessary referrals.

While telehealth provides opportunities to provide care for other pediatric visit types, this is not the case for well-child examinations. The preventive medicine service codes (99381-99397) require an "age-appropriate examination" which cannot be completed via telehealth. Additionally, immunizations are often administered at these visits. While there can be creative methods to provide preventive care, such as completing the components for the preventative service code (history, anticipatory guidance) via video and then having the child return to clinic for the examination and any vaccines, this creates multiple logistical challenges and potential errors. Various billing codes would be required. Patients who need examinations would need to be tracked, and these examinations would often be delayed from the initial history, making the correlation of prior history and physical poor. Additionally, history taking would likely be duplicated. Due to these requirements and challenges, well-child examinations are not conducted virtually. However, if a child is behind on their well-child visits and is seen virtually for another reason, providers should incorporate screening for emotional, social and behavioral concerns, age-appropriate surveillance and measurements, and provide age-appropriate anticipatory guidance. Particular attention should be given if concerns for neglect or abuse, as well as high-risk populations. These visits can provide a window into a child and family's daily routine and life not otherwise seen during an in-person visit.

Chronic Illness Management

Timely management of chronic pediatric illnesses such as allergies, migraines, and obesity is critical to providing optimal care. Pediatricians are concerned about the worsening of chronic conditions due to the COVID-19 pandemic and related stress. Prompt evaluation and management via telehealth of common issues such as migraines and asthma can provide timely care with avoidance of an urgent care or ER visit. Telehealth can also improve care coordination and management of chronic medical conditions by improving access to the patient's medical home. This can be conducted synchronously through virtual visits or asynchronously through remote monitoring and communication by the patient portal. Asynchronous telehealth applications such as the use of mobile devices or scheduled patient portal reminders can be used as medication reminders or to assist patients in recording and submitting clinical data.[12] Education can be provided via patient portal or other telehealth modality.

These measures can potentially improve patient follow-up rates and adherence to treatment plans leading to improved continuity of care, medical outcomes, and patient satisfaction (**Box 1**). In one study of children with asthma,[24] those with regular telehealth follow-ups, education, and medication prescription refills through telehealth resulted in fewer symptom days and ER visits. Furthermore, ER visits and hospitalizations were reduced by nearly half in those receiving telehealth intervention (7% vs 15%).[24]

> **Box 1**
> **Case 1**
>
> A 9 year old has mild persistent asthma. Asthma triggers include viral upper respiratory illnesses and allergic rhinitis. A video visit for asthma management was scheduled after it was noted that the family had requested frequent Albuterol refills. During the video visit, you ask the family to show you the child's inhalers. You discover that the family has been accidentally using the rescue asthma medication as the preventive asthma medication. You clarify for the family which asthma medication is preventive, which asthma medication is rescue and the indications for each. Family afterward can accurately demonstrate for you when they will use each asthma medication. You ask the patient to demonstrate the technique you learn that your patient has a spacer at home but is not using it. You review inhaler administration technique with the family and you are able to observe the patient practice using the spacer correctly. You are also able to review with the family interventions to try to reduce allergy triggers in the home such as the use of dust mite covers.

Injuries

Fractures and traumatic injuries were still commonplace, even during shut down and avoidance of organized activities and sports, early in the COVID-19 pandemic. While initial evaluation may need a hands-on examination, subsequent follow-ups can be conducted remotely. Over video, the patient and/or caregiver can palpate the area of previous injury and report if there is continued pain. Range of motion and functional testing, such as walking, jumping, and lifting objects, can be assessed and evaluated for pain or dysfunction. Additionally, providers can conduct telemedicine consultations with specialists such as orthopedists and rheumatologists who can help to determine the next steps including potential additional work up and if formal evaluation is necessary. This is particularly helpful in specialties whereby access is difficult.[12] Studies[25,26] have shown that when abnormalities are found on imaging or the ordering provider is uncertain of findings, remote radiography consultation for those with suspected fractures can reliably determine the next steps, including the need for surgical intervention and in-person orthopedic office visits (**Box 2**).

Mental Health

Psychiatry and mental health services were overburdened before the pandemic. Since the start of the pandemic, pediatricians and family physicians have been the initial resource for patients and also have provided ongoing mental health care for pediatric patients.

Pediatric patients needing care for mental health may require prompt evaluation and frequent follow-up, especially during times of urgency or crisis. Throughout the COVID-19 pandemic many children and adolescents have had difficulty coping with abrupt changes in their life, including the shutdown, transition to virtual school, hold on sports, fear and uncertainty of health, and loss of a parent(s), family, or friends. Mental health emergencies increased almost 25% for children 5 to 11 years of age and just more than 30% for those 12 to 17 years of age during March and October 2020. Suicide attempts increased more than 50% in adolescent teenage girls in 2021 compared with 2019.[27] Through telehealth, providers, and families may be able to access specialists and services. This is particularly important in locations whereby there are limited resources or oversaturation of psychiatric services. PCPs can consult with psychiatry when necessary. This approach can provide direct patient care, improving overall outcomes and provider and patient satisfaction. Busy families may be able to have more flexibility and access to engage with therapy services

Box 2
Case 2

A 12 year old suffers an inversion ankle injury while playing soccer and has immediate difficulty with ambulation. She subsequently develops worsening lateral ankle pain, swelling, and bruising. A video visit is initially scheduled. During this visit you assess her gait, which is antalgic. She has visible swelling and bruising on the lateral aspect of the ankle that extends down the lateral aspect of the foot. You assess her active range of motion, which is reduced. She is unable to get onto her toes and does not want to hop given pain. She points to the location of her pain as her lateral ankle, with reported tenderness over the lateral malleolus on self-palpation. With your instruction, she palpates the base of her 5th metatarsal, navicula, or the medial malleoli and reports no pain. No other pain in her foot. Given her mechanism, pain with walking, and limited examination, you decide to get standing ankle x-rays. On your review there are open growth plates (has not started menses). You think there is an irregularity of her physis and a bone fleck near the lateral malleolus seen on the lateral view. You are concerned about lateral ankle sprain with avulsion fracture and consult your sports medicine provider who reviews the images. They agree with your findings, recommend a tall cam walker and follow-up in the office.

virtually than previously in-person. Overall, telehealth can enhance the reach of mental health care to patients and pediatricians.[5]

Sexual Health

Telehealth can improve adolescent sexual health outcomes through educational and informative counseling as well as access to appointments with providers. Discussions regarding immunizations and safe sex practices can be conducted during telehealth visits.[5] One study[28] demonstrated that STI diagnosis and treatment, as well as partner notification, can be conducted virtually with outcomes equivalent to in-person visits. Attention must be made to patient confidentiality and safety during virtual visits. Using a private location, yes/no questions, thumbs up/down, or using a chat feature in the video visit platform can assist confidentiality.[10] The decision to examine genitalia virtually should be thoughtfully considered and potentially omitted or converted to an in-office visit. Photos submitted via patient portals are a permanent part of the patient's medical record. Additionally, a pediatric patient may not understand the important difference between allowing a virtual medical examination of the genitals and allowing inappropriate photos/videos to be taken of their genitals. For these reasons, if a genital examination is anticipated an in-office visit may be more appropriate.

Incorporating Learners

Telehealth will be a part of health care for the foreseeable future, and therefore requires strategies to teach learners how to manage the technical aspects of a telehealth encounter as it pertains to pediatric patients, especially in regard to the nuances of observation and parental involvement for a physical examination.[6,29] Over video we can assess a child's developmental milestones (**Box 3**), observe their home environment for safety, and watch them interact and participation in ADLs such, eating. Providing examples to learners during in-person encounters of how they could translate an examination into telehealth may be a helpful exercise. It is also important to remember that due to COVID-19 restrictions, many learners may have had fewer opportunities to perform well visits or practice their physical examination skills.

Future of Telehealth in Pediatrics

Technology will continue to advance and improve the patient and provider experience during a telehealth encounter. Additionally, telehealth offers flexibility for providers

---

Box 3
Case 3

A 3 year old girl was noted to have issues with constipation at her well-child examination. A follow-up video visit was scheduled 1 month later. Despite normal scores on developmental screens and lack of parental concerns about her development, you have had lingering worries about her because at all visits since she was 9 month old she cried uncontrollably and clung to her parents. She speaks a different language than you, so you cannot easily assess her language skills yourself. During the constipation video visit, you observe her in her home environment. She is happy, comfortable, and playful. She is eating a snack and eagerly shows you her toys. When she speaks, her mother interprets for you, and she demonstrates age-appropriate sentences and vocabulary.

---

with medical issues or restrictions unable to engage in in-person visits, office space constraints, and adjustments due to pandemics/endemics. For us to continue to meet the needs of our patients, there are some important items to consider.

We can continue to optimize telehealth experiences by evaluating and using remote patient monitoring, to take advantage of information many patients are already collecting from wearable fitness devices and clinical parameter tracking apps and devices. As telehealth will continue to be permanently integrated into medical care, it is necessary for future providers to receive adequate training in the field of telehealth. This should also include training on billing for telehealth. Telehealth training must be integrated into every level of medical education as well as regular continuing education for seasoned providers, so that providers can continue to be comfortable and adept with telehealth.

Changes made to billing and reimbursement during the COVID-19 PHE need to be made permanent. State licensing may benefit from more reciprocal arrangements between states, particularly those that share a border, so that access to care from your PCP is not limited to your current physical location.[16] Providers and offices need to continue to be aware of changing billing requirements.

SUMMARY

Although telehealth has been a part of medical care for more than 100 years, the COVID-19 pandemic propelled advancements in telehealth in the pediatric population. These advancements have given PCPs, pediatric specialists, and health extenders new ways to care for pediatric patients virtually. While well-child examinations are not currently appropriate for telehealth, both acute and chronic pediatric conditions are amenable to telehealth. A virtual encounter can save patients time and money, limit exposures to contagion, and improve their access to care. Pediatric providers are now appropriately billing for the various types of telehealth encounters. As we move forward with incorporating telehealth into our daily clinical practice, we can feel confident that properly used telehealth "is foundational to creating efficient, innovative, high-value care models in which patients get the right care at the right place at the right time, as well as investing in preventive care to reduce costly emergency department visits, all of which benefit all stakeholders in the health care system."[16]

CLINICS CARE POINTS

- Telehealth encompasses a wide variety of interactions with pediatric patients, their caregivers, and/or other providers including, but not limited to, video visits, portal messaging, and electronic consultations (E-consults).

- It is important to stay up to date on changing billing rules under the Public Health Emergency (PHE).
- Telehealth improves access to medical home and pediatric specialists.
- Appropriate pediatric telehealth visits can include behavioral health, developmental follow-up, follow-up of chronic conditions, minor illnesses, and some acute injuries.
- Inappropriate pediatric telehealth visits include the initial newborn examination, sensitive examination of the breasts or genitals, diagnoses that require a hands-on examination, and mental health visits whereby privacy cannot be guaranteed.
- If laboratories are expected for evidence-based medicine diagnosis and management, carefully consider if telehealth is truly the most appropriate visit type for your patient. If performed through telehealth, these visits could be improved by a hybrid model of initial video visits followed by laboratory testing.
- Pediatric care providers should familiarize themselves with appropriate reimbursement for all types of telehealth services, including portal messages and phone triage.
- Chronic illnesses may benefit from improved follow-up and management via various telehealth modalities.
- Telehealth training must be integrated into every level of medical education as well as regular continuing education for seasoned providers, so that providers can continue to be comfortable and adept with telehealth.

DISCLOSURE

The authors have nothing to disclose.

REFERENCES

1. The Chartis Group. Telehealth adoption tracker. 2021. Available at: https://reports.chartis.com/telehealth_trends_and_implications-2021/. Accessed November 23, 2021.
2. The Chartis Group. What the COVID-19 telehealth spike revealed about achieving lasting adoption of virtual care. 2021. Available at: https://www.chartis.com/virtual-care-article-1. Accessed November 23, 2021.
3. Koonin LM, Hoots B, Tsang CA, et al. Trends in the use of telehealth during the emergence of the COVID-19 pandemic - United States, January-March 2020. MMWR Morb Mortal Wkly Rep 2020;69(43):1595–9. Erratum in: MMWR Morb Mortal Wkly Rep. 2020 Nov 13;69(45):1711.
4. The Chartis Group. Tracking U.S. telehealth adoption a year Into the COVID-19 pandemic: trend analysis & implications for health systems. 2021. Available at: https://reports.chartis.com/telehealth_trends_and_implications-2021/. Accessed January 11, 2022.
5. Tomines A. Pediatric telehealth: approaches by specialty and implications for general pediatric care. Adv Pediatr 2019;66:55–85.
6. American Academy of Pediatrics. Guidance on the necessary use of telehealth during the COVID-19 pandemic. 2022. Available at: https://www.aap.org/en/pages/2019-novel-coronavirus-covid-19-infections/clinical-guidance/guidance-on-the-necessary-use-of-telehealth-during-the-covid-19-pandemic/. Accessed January 23, 2022.
7. Centers for Medicare and Medicaid Services. Medicare wellness visits. Available at: https://www.cms.gov/Outreach-and-Education/Medicare-Learning-Network-

MLN/MLNProducts/preventive-services/medicare-wellness-visits.html. Accessed January, 22, 2022.

8. U.S. Department of Health and Human Services. Public health emergency. Updated April 2021. Available at: https://www.phe.gov/emergency/news/healthactions/phe/Pages/COVID-15April2021.aspx. Accessed December 12, 2021.

9. Telehealth.HHS.gov. HIPAA flexibility for telehealth technology. 2021. Available at: https://telehealth.hhs.gov/providers/policy-changes-during-the-covid-19-public-health-emergency/. Accessed November 16, 2021.

10. Curfman A, McSwain SD, Chuo J, et al. Pediatric telehealth in the COVID-19 pandemic era and beyond. Pediatrics 2021;148(3). e2020047795.

11. U.S. Department of Health and Human Services. Renewal of determination that a public health emergency exists. 2022. Available at: https://aspr.hhs.gov/legal/PHE/Pages/COVID19-12Apr2022.aspx. Accessed April 14, 2022.

12. Taylor L, Portnoy JM. Telemedicine for general pediatrics. Pediatr Ann 2019; 48(12):e479–84.

13. McSwain SD, Bernard J, Burke BL Jr, et al. American telemedicine association operating procedures for pediatric telehealth. Telemed J E Health 2017;23(9): 699–706.

14. Foster CB, Martinez KA, Sabella C, et al. Patient satisfaction and antibiotic prescribing for respiratory infections by telemedicine. Pediatrics 2019;144(3): e20190844.

15. Fiks AG, Jenssen BP, Ray KN. A Defining moment for pediatric primary care telehealth. JAMA Pediatr 2021;175(1):9–10.

16. Curfman AL, Hackell JM, Herendeen NE, et al. Section on telehealth care, committee on practice and ambulatory medicine, committee on pediatric workforce. telehealth: improving access to and quality of pediatric health care. Pediatrics 2021;148(3). e2021053129.

17. Hooshmand M, Yao K. Challenges facing children with special healthcare needs and their families: telemedicine as a bridge to care. Telemed J E Health 2017; 23(1):18–24.

18. Marcin JP, Ellis J, Mawis R, et al. Using telemedicine to provide pediatric subspecialty care to children with special health care needs in an underserved rural community. Pediatrics 2004;113(1 Pt 1):1–6.

19. Sisk B, Alexander J, Bodnar C, et al. Pediatrician attitudes toward and experiences with telehealth use: Results From a National Survey. Acad Pediatr 2020; 20(5):628–35.

20. Johnson TM, Sikora K, Reilly K, et al. Telehealth in primary care: meeting patient and family needs. Pediatr 2021;147(3_MeetingAbstract):985–6.

21. Rea CJ, Wenren LM, Tran KD, et al. Shared care: using an electronic consult form to facilitate primary care provider-specialty care coordination. Acad Pediatr 2018; 18(7):797–804.

22. Ray KN, Shi Z, Gidengil CA, et al. Antibiotic prescribing during pediatric direct-to-consumer telemedicine visits. Pediatrics 2019;143(5):e20182491.

23. McConnochie KM, Conners GP, Brayer AF, et al. Differences in diagnosis and treatment using telemedicine versus in-person evaluation of acute illness. Ambul Pediatr 2006;6(4):187–95, discussion 196-7.

24. Halterman JS, Fagnano M, Tajon RS, et al. Effect of the school-based telemedicine enhanced asthma management (SBTEAM) Program on asthma morbidity: a randomized clinical trial. JAMA Pediatr 2018;172(3):e174938.

25. Goost H, Witten J, Heck A, et al. Image and diagnosis quality of x-ray image transmission via cell phone camera: a project study evaluating quality and reliability. PLoS One 2012;7(10):e43402.

26. Zennaro F, Grosso D, Fascetta R, et al. Teleradiology for remote consultation using iPad improves the use of health system human resources for paediatric fractures: prospective controlled study in a tertiary care hospital in Italy. BMC Health Serv Res 2014;14(1):327.

27. HealthyChildren.org from the AAP. . Mental health during COVID-19: signs your child may need more support. 2021. Available at: https://www.healthychildren.org/English/health-issues/conditions/COVID-19/Pages/Signs-your-Teen-May-Need-More-Support.aspx. Accessed January 14, 2022.

28. Aicken CRH, Sutcliffe LJ, Gibbs J, et al. Using the esexual health clinic to access chlamydia treatment and care via the internet: a qualitative interview study sexually transmitted. Infections 2018;94:241–7.

29. Alcocer Alkureishi M, Lenti G, Choo ZY, et al. Teaching telemedicine: the next frontier for medical educators. JMIR Med Educ 2021;7(2):e29099.

Telehealth Considerations for the Adolescent Patient

Laura Heinrich, MD[a,b,1], Anita K. Hernandez, MD[a,*], Anna R. Laurie, MD[a]

KEYWORDS

- Adolescent medicine/AYA/Young adult • Telehealth/telemedicine/virtual care
- Confidentiality • Inclusive care

KEY POINTS

- The use of telehealth for the care of adolescent and young adult (AYA) populations is growing in popularity, given the changing health care landscape and the needs of patients.
- Physicians and providers implementing telehealth for adolescents need to provide structure for confidentiality, access to health information, and interdisciplinary support.
- AYA can be safely counseled on and prescribed contraception using clinical criteria that reliably exclude the possibility of pregnancy.
- Delivery via telehealth of certain services such as the evaluation and treatment of eating disorders, gender-affirming hormone therapy, and treatment of substance use disorders can help to expand these services to AYA who may otherwise through geography or for reasons of lack of access to transportation be unable to access these services.

BACKGROUND

The use of telehealth for the treatment of adolescent and young adult (AYA) populations has been described for several years, and the SARS-CoV2 pandemic rapidly transformed the landscape of care. The opportunities for the implementation of telehealth for AYAs are many. The following will present a review of the evolving best practices, evidence, and expert opinions.

SETTING AND SET-UP

To perform virtual visits with adolescents, there must be a platform to conduct the visit in a confidential manner. Many electronic health record (EHR) systems have a video

[a] Department of Family Medicine, University of Michigan, 1801 Briarwood Circle Building 10, Ann Arbor, MI 48108, USA; [b] Virtual Care Department, University of Michigan Health, Ann Arbor, MI, USA
[1] Present address: 200 Arnet Street Suite 200, Ypsilanti, MI 48198.
* Corresponding author.
E-mail address: akhernan@med.umich.edu

Prim Care Clin Office Pract 49 (2022) 597–607
https://doi.org/10.1016/j.pop.2022.04.006
0095-4543/22/© 2022 Elsevier Inc. All rights reserved.

product embedded, which allows access for adolescents.[1] However, AYA access to the platform may be limited due to restrictions to the system for minors. Some medical practices or institutions may have a virtual platform separate from the EMR which provides the patient access through a link sent via text message or email. Despite attempts at confidentiality, one study demonstrated that more than half of adolescent accounts were estimated to have been accessed by guardians at least once.[2] The creation of proxy accounts for the guardian provides limited views, although, in the aforementioned study, guardians bypassed these proxy accounts. We recommend consulting with your practice or institutional information technology specialists, or EMR vendor to ensure capabilities exist to allow proxy accounts for minors.

The Society for Adolescent Health and Medicine (SAHM) has set recommendations for the use of the EHR for AYA, and experts in health informatics have described potential approaches.[3,4] SAHM states that "EHRs should have the functionality to provide access to information via the patient portal to parents while also allowing for flexibility in the protection of confidential health information." See **Table 1** for options on how to best set up the portal access.

Care provided through telehealth should be analogous to what is available in-person, with parity across patient characteristics and demographics. Other services necessary for patient care should be available, including interpreter services and staff needed for patient and family education, safety reporting, and so forth. In a study within an adolescent medicine clinic, 85% of respondents found telehealth easy to use; though many (one-quarter of AYA and one-third of caregivers) experienced technical problems.[5] Telehealth in the setting of the patient-centered medical home provides continuity and comprehensiveness unique from independent third-party health care providers.

In a national study of over one thousand primary care physicians who serve adolescents, 89% reported using telehealth, with most of the respondents agreeing that adolescent use of telehealth increases access to care.[6]

Most telehealth for adolescent patients is delivered through primary care and psychiatry office-based settings; however, there is increased utilization in specialty care. School-based health centers (SBHC) used telehealth even before the COVID-19 pandemic.[7] SBHCs using telehealth were more likely to serve rural communities than those not using telehealth, highlighting that telehealth has promise in delivering care to areas with scarce health provider resources. However, telehealth exclusive SBHCs were less likely to use a multidisciplinary approach compared with traditional models, such as the inclusion of a behavioral health professional. The models used in SBHCs can be expanded into primary care practices.

USE CASES

The potential use conditions for telehealth in the adolescent patient is broad, including those specific to adolescent patients as well as acute and chronic conditions seen in the general primary care office.

Mental Health

Telepsychiatry has been the most widely used application in the adolescent population.[8] Demand for mental health care increased in the United States, even before the pandemic. In adult populations, most antidepressants are prescribed by their primary care provider.[9] Between 2007 and 2010, approximately 48% of adolescent mental health office visits were seen by psychiatry.[10]

Table 1 Potential access to EHR of adolescents, 13–17 years old			
	Nonconfidential	**Confidential**	**Considerations**
Option 1	Patient & Guardian	No access	Information parity
Option 2	Patient & Guardian	Patient	Patient can customize the portal
Option 3	Patient & Guardian	Patient & Guardian	Special patient cases, for example, cognitive impairment or cancer
Option 4	No access	No access	

Data from Society for Adolescent Health and Medicine, Gray SH, Pasternak RH, et al. Recommendations for electronic health record use for delivery of adolescent health care. J Adolesc Health. 2014;54(4):487-490.

Attention deficit hyperactivity disorder

The treatment of attention deficit hyperactivity disorder (ADHD) has been evaluated in the virtual setting, although there has not been a comprehensive evaluation of care via virtual means outside of specialty care.[11] The primary care physician can provide the follow-up and treatment of ADHD virtually or use a hybrid model of both in-person and video visits. The EMR can be used to collect collateral information from parents or patients via questionnaires, or parents can upload teacher information via the patient portal for a comprehensive assessment. A challenge can be routine monitoring of objective data, particularly during important growth periods of adolescence. The practice should consider how to provide adequate monitoring of vital signs and weight velocity if the patient is on stimulant medication with either in-person visits or the use of patient-reported data.

Depression and anxiety

In 2017, an estimated 3.2 million adolescents aged 12 to 17 in the United States had at least one major depressive episode,[12] and this number increased amidst the SARS-CoV-2 pandemic. According to a national poll, 1 in 3 teen girls and 1 in 5 teen boys have experienced new or worsening anxiety since March 2020.[13] In 2020, there was a more than 30% increase in emergency room visits for mental health in those between 12 and 17.[14] The evaluation and treatment of depression and anxiety can be performed virtually and has been well studied for feasibility and satisfaction. In a study of 172 youth and 387 visits over 1 year, parents indicated high levels of satisfaction with telepsychiatry, and this satisfaction increased with return appointments. However, in that same study, parents tended toward higher satisfaction with younger children as opposed to adolescents.[15]

Like the provision of telehealth as a whole, it is important to optimize the setting for the authenticity and replication of the in-person experience, through "webside" manner.[16] This can be achieved with a variety of techniques involving nonverbal techniques or room or background layout, such as maintaining good posture, gestures that fall within the camera screen, and making sure to take pauses while speaking to allow time for a response if there is a transmission delay. This highlights the importance of rapport building and confidentiality. Seager and colleagues[17] developed tips for building rapport with youth, including maintaining gaze at the camera, using gestures such as high 5 or thumbs up, allowing the adolescent to share a personal interest or item with you, and having the adolescent have control in choosing the telehealth background feature.

The clinician and medical practice should have policies and procedures in place to respond to acute safety concerns. If a patient discloses intent to harm themselves or others, immediate action should be taken. The University of Michigan Health System has created scripting and resources to be used if a patient were to express thoughts of harming themself or others, which includes the contact information for the local psychiatric emergency services, instructions on calling emergency medical services (EMS) when necessary, and regional and national hotlines.

Eating disorders

Primary care physicians play a significant role in the detection and treatment of eating disorders in adolescents.[18,19] Models of family-based therapy for the treatment of eating disorders have been successfully delivered via telehealth, through the use of family educational modules and family therapy delivered via videoconferencing over regular, phased follow-up with therapists, families, and patients in a structured program.[20] As care was rapidly transitioned to telehealth during the COVID-19 pandemic, one study demonstrated that individuals with eating disorders appreciated the availability of telehealth, while 47% of US respondents and 74% of respondents from the Netherlands perceived the quality of their care was worse than what they had received previously face-to-face. It was noted that this survey was performed early in the pandemic as providers were just starting to use telehealth platforms.[21] In a review of literature evaluating the impact of the COVID-19 pandemic on the treatment of eating disorders, albeit with small sample sizes, 3 studies found the use of telehealth to be safe, tolerated and effective for improving general mental health and eating disorder symptoms.[22] The care of patients with eating disorders is typically multidisciplinary, a format which can be converted to virtual delivery including options for group videos with practitioners and patients alike.

Substance use

Telehealth has rapidly expanded for the treatment of substance use disorders with the COVID-19 pandemic. At the end of March 2020, the Drug Enforcement Administration (DEA) published a policy regarding the prescription of controlled substances during the ongoing COVID-19 Public Health Emergency. This allowed for the expanded use of telehealth services for substance use disorders (SUD), specifically noting that patients establishing care for the treatment of opioid use disorder (OUD) could be evaluated via telephone or two-way audio-visual communication.[23] In June 2020, the Substance Abuse and Mental Health Services Administration (SAMHSA) along with the Centers for Medicare and Medicaid Services (CMS) advised that insurers cover substance abuse services provided on telehealth and remote platforms and advised strongly that substance use services be uninterrupted during the pandemic.[24]

Several systems have been providing substance use telehealth services and have published their preliminary experiences. In 2018, a study examined claims data between 2010 and 2017 from a large commercial insurer which included data from patients as young as 12. It found patients accessing telehealth for their SUD were more likely to be in rural areas, more likely to have a more severe SUD diagnosis and a concurrent diagnosis of mental illness, and more likely to be in upper income quartiles.[25] The University of California at San Francisco Health System gained experience with the use of telehealth for the addiction treatment of AYA with their established addiction program, initially in the care of established patients and then for new patients starting in March 2020.[26] An audio-visual platform was used both for federally required intake interviews and for visits with clinicians. Adolescents and their parents were also encouraged to log on from different devices in different, private locations to provide confidentiality. Buprenorphine inductions were planned and conducted virtually with the help of a youth identified support person. Outcomes were not known at the time of publication and potential challenges include lack of private or safe space to perform a telehealth visit, changing national guidelines and permissions for the provision of substance use care via telehealth, and provider discomfort with providing these types of visits virtually.

Although we have mounting evidence that substance abuse care can be delivered virtually, it remains unclear how AYA would prefer to have their care delivered. A survey of just more than 400 AYA receiving mental health and substance abuse services in Ontario, Canada concluded that youth, in general, seem willing to engage in virtual delivery of care, but have concerns about privacy, confidentiality, and are more willing to engage in individual services than group services.[27]

Gender-affirming care

About 2% of high school age youth identify as transgender.[28] Provision of gender-affirming care to transgender and nonbinary youth is uniquely suited to virtual care given the wide geographic variation in the availability of gender-affirming care. Many providers who traditionally offer pediatric and adolescent gender-affirming care and prescribe hormone therapy practice in large academic centers. In addition, many AYA do not have adequate access to transportation to independently access in-person services. Furthermore, gender nonconforming youth require not only spaces of care in which they feel validated and welcomed for their primary care but also access to gender-affirming care, hormones, and gender-affirming procedures. Though there are spaces that provide both primary care and gender-affirming hormone therapy to transgender youth, AYA frequently need to seek care in more than one location.

A 2020 survey of transgender youth demonstrated that many expressed interest in receiving care through virtual means, and those desiring telehealth services were more likely to have lower perceived parental support ($P = .001$).[29] This is particularly important as youth with lower parental support are also more likely to experience mental health problems.

Not only would the use of telehealth services expand access to gender-affirming care for at-risk youth, specifically encouraging primary care practices that already provide gender-affirming care to use telehealth could expand access to those most at risk. Personal author experience at an AYA health center has shown that with the initiation of telehealth services during the COVID-19 pandemic, the number of transgender AYAs served both for primary care and for gender-affirming hormone care increased significantly, with many patients establishing care through telehealth who would have otherwise traveled 2 to 3 hours to the health center. Follow-up care and show rate has also been more reliable. Pitfalls have included maintenance of a private space to discuss gender-affirming services, continued lack of parental support for gender-affirming care, and difficulty with the coordination of laboratory draws and laboratory services from a distance.

Contraception and reproductive health

Reproductive health care, an essential facet of medical care, can be safely and satisfactorily provided via numerous telehealth modalities for AYA populations.[30] A study of adult patients who received contraception counseling in the early pandemic showed that 86% of survey respondents were very satisfied with telehealth, and 51% preferred it to an in-person visit. Privacy was cited as a major concern, particularly with video visits, and some patients expressed a preference for phone visits for this reason. With AYA populations confidentiality is a major consideration for satisfaction with reproductive health discussions conducted via telehealth.[31] Compared with in-person visits, there is clearly a limitation in the extent of options that can be offered at the time of the visit. Any procedural contraceptives (IUDs, implants) or injectable contraceptives can be discussed but not completed, which presents an opportunity for a patient to be lost to follow-up. Many patients will continue to feel more comfortable with the privacy afforded by in-person visits. Still, in the wake of the COVID-19 pandemic, the American College of Obstetricians and Gynecologists (ACOG) suggests that contraceptive prescribing and counseling, routine medical abortion care, and asymptomatic ovarian cyst management should be conducted preferentially by virtual means.[32]

As laws vary by state as to what an individual under the age of 18 can consent to for contraception, testing and treatment of sexually transmitted infections (STI), pregnancy care, and pregnancy termination, it is crucial to be familiar with your own region's laws before providing this care directly to adolescents both in-person and with telemedicine. The Guttmacher Institute provides a summary here: https://www. guttmacher.org/state-policy/explore/overview-minors-consent-law.[33]

Contraceptive counseling and prescribing are quite amenable to telehealth, as no pelvic or other physical examination is necessary before prescribing hormonal contraception. Thorough medical history, with the review of contraindications and medical eligibility, along with a recent blood pressure measurement is sufficient to safely prescribe, and providing care via telehealth can reduce barriers to this important care.[34] The Centers for Disease Control and Prevention (CDC) has published extensive medical eligibility criteria to review patient criteria and medical history in choosing safe contraceptive options, such as reproductive history, history of chronic disease, concurrent infections, drug interactions and more. The CDC also provides highly accurate (negative predictive value 99%–100%) criteria to be reasonably sure a patient is not pregnant; if she has no signs or symptoms of pregnancy and meets any of the following, a health care provider can be reasonably sure she is not pregnant:

- Is ≤ 7 days after the start of normal menses
- Has not had sexual intercourse as the start of last normal menses
- Has been correctly and consistently using a reliable method of contraception
- Is ≤ 7 days after spontaneous or induced abortion
- Is within 4 weeks postpartum
- Is fully or nearly fully breastfeeding (exclusively breastfeeding or the vast majority [≥85%] of feeds are breastfeeds), amenorrheic, and less than 6 months postpartum

Urine pregnancy testing, either by home test or a sample transported to a nearby laboratory, can be conducted for additional evaluation but is not necessary for every patient, and must be considered in terms of other patient factors such as last menstrual period, timing of last intercourse, and recent pregnancy. If uncertainty remains regarding the possibility of pregnancy, the benefits still outweigh the risks of beginning or recommending contraception during a telehealth visit (with the exception of IUD insertion) and following up with a pregnancy test 2 to 4 weeks later.[35]

Aside from providing contraceptive prescriptions, extensive counseling can be conducted for long-acting reversible contraceptives (LARC), barrier and nonhormonal methods, emergency contraception, and contraception following pregnancy or pregnancy loss/termination. Similar counseling is also translatable to the discussion and management of common menstrual problems including menorrhagia, dysmenorrhea, polycystic ovarian syndrome, and so forth. While there currently are no specifically defined thresholds for suggesting in-person evaluation for these conditions, we suggest using clinical judgment and considering the same above medical eligibility criteria and pregnancy rule-out criteria used for the initiation of contraception, and ensuring there are no red flag symptoms that would necessitate in-person examination or further testing with ultrasound or laboratory evaluation.

Sexually transmitted infections are a massive public health issue, costing the US health care system billions of dollars yearly, with almost one-half of new infections occurring in AYA between the ages of 15 to 24.[36] Telehealth provides a low-barrier way to discuss prevention and screening for STI, in addition to providing treatment to patients from self-collected samples when accessible, and partner treatment whereby allowed by law. Accurate testing may be limited by the ability of a patient to self-test, which requires access to a clinic or laboratory and may be limited by the availability and acceptability of different testing modalities (ie, urethral or vaginal swab, urine, or blood testing), which could more easily be obtained during an in-person visit. Telehealth is also not sufficient for all STI treatment, as some conditions necessitate intramuscular administration of antibiotics. Prescribing preexposure prophylaxis (PrEP) for HIV via telehealth may be an important factor in improving uptake and adherence to PrEP, although further studies need to be conducted to evaluate this in the adult and AYA population.[37,38]

A full discussion of prenatal care or pregnancy termination provision via telehealth is outside the scope of this article; however, the ACOG Committee Opinion describes comparable perinatal outcomes and improved patient satisfaction with virtual prenatal care.[39] Acknowledging vast differences in legal barriers and FDA limitations to pregnancy termination, direct-to-patient telehealth services have been found to be similarly safe and effective compared with in-clinic management of medical termination; patient satisfaction and acceptance are also high with telehealth.[40]

CONFIDENTIALITY

The American Academy of Family Physicians (AAFP), along with the American Academy of Pediatrics (AAP), and SAHM endorse the confidential care for adolescent patients.[41–43] Maintaining confidentiality and privacy is of paramount importance while conducting virtual care to allow for complete health care and to foster independence within the health care system. As with in-person care, the health care provider should be familiar with regional laws and institutional policies as they relate to adolescent care and should be familiar with EMR system procedures for adolescent and parent proxy access to the patient portal, open notes, results, and ability to access virtual visits if embedded within the EMR.

The health care provider should create a safe and comfortable environment for both adolescents and parents by reviewing the limits of confidentiality and consent with all telehealth and be aware of special circumstances such as emancipated minors, foster status, legal guardianship, and custody agreements. Care should always be taken to ensure Health Insurance Portability and Accountability Act of 1996 (HIPAA) standards are met to protect adolescent Protected Health Information (PHI) by using private space to conduct virtual visits whenever possible and be cognizant of the patient's environment as well, adjusting your discussion as needed to ensure their privacy as best able in the circumstances if you cannot verify who may see or hear the conversation. In a study of adolescents and caregivers, there was divergence in acceptability of telehealth with regard to perceived privacy between the patient and caregiver, with a significantly higher proportion of AYA rating telehealth as inferior to in-person care.[5] In addition, in academic settings when learners are present, it is possible that an adolescent may be sharing information with more individuals than they realize and clinical encounters should be aware of ensuring adolescents are aware of their providers with a clear introduction of who may be a learner.

Updates regarding HIPAA flexibility due to COVID-19 can be found here as changes evolve with the pandemic: https://www.hhs.gov/hipaa/for-professionals/special-topics/hipaa-covid19/index.html.

LEGAL IMPLICATIONS AND BILLING

Like adult telehealth services, health care providers should verify malpractice coverage for telehealth and confirm licensing regulations based on the location whereby adolescent health services are to be provided. Providers should obtain informed consent regarding rights, responsibilities, and expectations, including limitations of virtual care in accordance with local laws and institutional policy.

While subject to change in time, location, and payer, reimbursement for services provided via covered synchronous telemedicine services (phone, video visits) is currently on par with in-person encounters. CPT codes for routine office visits performed with telemedicine can be used with modifier GT or 95. Telephone codes 99441 (5–10 minutes), 99,442 (11–20 minutes), and 99,443 (20–30 minutes) may now also be used. Modifier GQ is also available for asynchronous telecommunications. For further reference, the Center for Connected Health Policy maintains a database of telehealth policies, laws, and regulations at the federal and state levels here: https://www.cchpca.org/all-telehealth-policies/.

We recommend consulting with your local experts for practice, institutional, or state requirements given the rapidity with which the current guidelines may change, particularly in light of the Public Health Emergency (PHE) and the potential for changing guidelines and regulations in the coming months. During the PHE, covered health care providers may communicate through noncompliant technologies, provided there are no public-facing privacy risks, with more guidance here https://www.hhs.gov/hipaa/for-professionals/special-topics/emergency-preparedness/notification-enforcement-discretion-telehealth/index.html.

SUMMARY

Recent experience with the rapid expansion of telehealth has shown that it is a viable and often preferred means to deliver health care to adolescent patients. Health care providers and patients with AYA and families have generally had high degrees of satisfaction with the use of telehealth.[44] Common use cases include the treatment of mental health and substance use disorders as well as acute care. Opportunity exists to study telehealth for anticipatory guidance, education, and counseling on topics including vaccine hesitancy or with ongoing management of chronic diseases in AYA populations. Barriers to providing care include the ability to ensure and maintain confidentiality, adolescent access to patient health portal, among others. State-to-state variability in minor consent laws makes larger scale guidelines and recommendations for the delivery of confidential care challenging. Health care providers and practices are encouraged to implement comprehensive services for adolescent patients, which should include the provision of telehealth options.

CLINICS CARE POINTS

- Providers should be familiar with their local minor consent and confidentiality laws when providing telehealth services to adolescent patients.

- Practices that provide specialty care to adolescents and young adults such as gender-affirming care or care of substance use disorders should consider telehealth as a means of expanding access to those services.
- Adolescents and young adults can be safely prescribed contraception through virtual care without a clinic pregnancy test with the use of validated clinical criteria for excluding a pregnancy.
- Though adolescents and young adults may find it easy to connect to telehealth services, it should not be assumed that telehealth is their preferred model of care.

DISCLOSURE

The authors have nothing to disclose.

REFERENCES

1. Carlson JL, Goldstein R. Using the electronic health record to conduct adolescent telehealth visits in the time of COVID-19. J Adolesc Health 2020;67(2):157–8.
2. Ip W, Yang S, Parker J, et al. Assessment of prevalence of adolescent patient portal account access by guardians. JAMA Netw Open 2021;4(9):e2124733.
3. Gray SH, Pasternak RH, Gooding HC, et al. Recommendations for electronic health record use for delivery of adolescent health care. J Adolesc Health 2014;54(4):487–90.
4. Bourgeois FC, Taylor PL, Emans SJ, et al. Whose personal control? creating private, personally controlled health records for pediatric and adolescent patients. J Am Med Inform Assoc 2008;15(6):737–43.
5. Wood SM, Pickel J, Phillips AW, et al. Acceptability, feasibility, and quality of telehealth for adolescent health care delivery during the COVID-19 pandemic: cross-sectional study of patient and family experiences. JMIR Pediatr Parent 2021;4(4): e32708.
6. Gilkey MB, Kong WY, Huang Q, et al. Using telehealth to deliver primary care to adolescents during and after the COVID-19 pandemic: national survey study of us primary care professionals. J Med Internet Res 2021;23(9):e31240.
7. Love H, Panchal N, Schlitt J, et al. The use of telehealth in school-based health centers. Glob Pediatr Health 2019;6. https://doi.org/10.1177/2333794X19884194.
8. Paing WW, Weller RA, Welsh B, et al. Telemedicine in children and adolescents. Curr Psychiatry Rep 2009;11(2):114–9.
9. Mojtabai R, Olfson M. National patterns in antidepressant treatment by psychiatrists and general medical providers: results from the national comorbidity survey replication. J Clin Psychiatry 2008;69(7):1064–74.
10. Olfson M, Kroenke K, Wang S, et al. Trends in office-based mental health care provided by psychiatrists and primary care physicians. J Clin Psychiatry 2014; 75(3):21732.
11. Spencer T, Noyes E, Biederman J. Telemedicine in the Management of ADHD: Literature Review of Telemedicine in ADHD. J Atten Disord 2020;24(1):3–9.
12. Results from the 2017 National Survey on Drug Use and Health: Detailed Tables, SAMHSA, CBHSQ. Available at: https://www.samhsa.gov/data/sites/default/files/cbhsq-reports/NSDUHDetailedTabs2017/NSDUHDetailedTabs2017.htm#tab8-56A. Accessed July 7, 2021.
13. Freed GL, Singer DC, Gebremariam A, Schultz SL, Clark SJ. How the pandemic has impacted teen mental health. C.S. Mott Children's Hospital National Poll on

Children's Health, University of Michigan. Vol 38, Issue 2, March 2021. Available at: https://mottpoll.org/reports/how-pandemic-has-impacted-teen-mental-health.

14. Leeb RT. Mental health–related emergency department visits among children aged 18 years during the COVID-19 pandemic — United States, January 1–October 17, 2020. MMWR Morb Mortal Wkly Rep 2020;69. https://doi.org/10.15585/mmwr.mm6945a3.

15. Myers KM, Valentine JM, Melzer SM. Child and adolescent telepsychiatry: utilization and satisfaction. Telemed J E Health 2008;14(2):131–7.

16. Roth DE, Ramtekkar U, Zeković-Roth S. Telepsychiatry. Child Adolesc Psychiatr Clin N Am 2019;28(3):377–95.

17. Seager van Dyk I, Kroll J, Martinez R, et al. COVID-19 tips: building rapport with youth via telehealth. 2020. https://doi.org/10.13140/RG.2.2.23293.10727.

18. Williams PM, Goodie J, Motsinger CD. Treating eating disorders in primary care. Am Fam Physician 2008;77(2):187–95.

19. Lebow J, Mattke A, Narr C, et al. Can adolescents with eating disorders be treated in primary care? A retrospective clinical cohort study. J Eat Disord 2021;9(1):55.

20. Anderson KE, Byrne C, Goodyear A, et al. Telemedicine of family-based treatment for adolescent anorexia nervosa: a protocol of a treatment development study. J Eat Disord 2015;3:25.

21. Termorshuizen JD, Watson HJ, Thornton LM, et al. Early impact of COVID-19 on individuals with self-reported eating disorders: a survey of 1,000 individuals in the United States and the Netherlands. Int J Eat Disord 2020;53(11):1780–90.

22. Linardon J, Messer M, Rodgers RF, et al. A systematic scoping review of research on COVID-19 impacts on eating disorders: a critical appraisal of the evidence and recommendations for the field. Int J Eat Disord. n/a(n/a). doi:10.1002/eat.23640.

23. COVID-19 Information Page. Available at: https://www.deadiversion.usdoj.gov/coronavirus.html. Accessed December 2, 2021.

24.. Centers for Medicare & Medicaid Services (CMS) and Substance Abuse, Mental Health Services Administration (SAMHSA), Leveraging Existing Health and Disease Management Programs to Provide Mental Health and Substance Use Disorder Resources During the COVID-19 Public Health, Emergency, (PHE)1., 3 https://www.cms.gov/CCIIO/Programs-and-Initiatives/Health-Insurance-Marketplaces/Downloads/Mental-Health-Substance-Use-Disorder-Resources-COVID-19.pdf.

25. Huskamp HA, Busch AB, Souza J, et al. How Is telemedicine being used in opioid and other substance use disorder treatment? Health Aff Proj Hope 2018;37(12):1940–7.

26. Barney A, Buckelew S, Mesheriakova V, et al. The COVID-19 pandemic and rapid implementation of adolescent and young adult telemedicine: challenges and opportunities for innovation. J Adolesc Health 2020;67(2):164–71.

27. Hawke LD, Sheikhan NY, MacCon K, et al. Going virtual: youth attitudes toward and experiences of virtual mental health and substance use services during the COVID-19 pandemic. BMC Health Serv Res 2021;21(1):340.

28. Rider GN, McMorris BJ, Gower AL, et al. Health and care utilization of transgender and gender nonconforming youth: a population-based study. Pediatrics 2018;141(3):e20171683.

29. Sequeira GM, Kidd KM, Coulter RWS, et al. Transgender youths' perspectives on telehealth for delivery of gender-affirming care. J Adolesc Health 2020. https://doi.org/10.1016/j.jadohealth.2020.08.028.

30. Wilkinson TA, Kottke MJ, Berlan ED. Providing contraception for young people during a pandemic is essential health care. JAMA Pediatr 2020;174(9):823–4.
31. Stifani BM, Smith A, Avila K, et al. Telemedicine for contraceptive counseling: Patient experiences during the early phase of the COVID-19 pandemic in New York City. Contraception 2021;104(3):254–61.
32. COVID-19 FAQs for obstetrician-gynecologists, obstetrics. Available at: https://www.acog.org/en/clinical-information/physician-faqs/covid-19-faqs-for-ob-gyns-obstetrics. Accessed December 13, 2021.
33. An overview of consent to reproductive health services by young people. Guttmacher Institute; 2016. Available at: https://www.guttmacher.org/state-policy/explore/overview-minors-consent-law. Accessed February 1, 2022.
34. Lesnewski R, Prine L. Initiating hormonal contraception. Am Fam Physician 2006; 74(1):105–12.
35. Curtis KM. U.S. Medical eligibility criteria for contraceptive use, 2016. MMWR Recomm Rep 2016;65.
36. STI incidence, prevalence, cost estimates | CDC. 2021. Available at: https://www.cdc.gov/nchhstp/newsroom/2021/2018-STI-incidence-prevalence-estimates.html. Accessed December 13, 2021.
37. Edeza A, Karina Santamaria E, Valente PK, et al. Experienced barriers to adherence to pre-exposure prophylaxis for HIV prevention among MSM: a systematic review and meta-ethnography of qualitative studies. AIDS Care 2021;33(6): 697–705.
38. Velloza J, Kapogiannis B, Bekker LG, et al. Interventions to improve daily medication use among adolescents and young adults: what can we learn for youth pre-exposure prophylaxis services? AIDS Lond Engl 2021;35(3):463–75.
39. Implementing telehealth in practice: ACOG committee opinion summary, number 798. Obstet Gynecol 2020;135(2):493–4.
40. Telemedicine for medication abortion - PubMed. Available at: https://pubmed.ncbi.nlm.nih.gov/31356771/. Accessed December 13, 2021.
41. Adolescent Health Care. Confidentiality. Available at: https://www.aafp.org/about/policies/all/adolescent-confidentiality.html. Accessed May 5, 2021.
42. Confidentiality in adolescent health care: ACOG committee opinion, number 803. Obstet Gynecol 2020;135(4):e171.
43. Ford C, English A, Sigman G. Confidential health care for adolescents: position paper of the Society for Adolescent Medicine. J Adolesc Health 2004;35(2): 160–7.
44. Tully L, Case L, Arthurs N, et al. Barriers and facilitators for implementing paediatric telemedicine: rapid review of user perspectives. Front Pediatr 2021;9: 630365.

Prenatal Care via Telehealth

Alison Shmerling, MD, MPH*, Molly Hoss, MD, Naomi Malam, MD,
Elizabeth W. Staton, MSTC, Corey Lyon, DO

KEYWORDS

- Telehealth • Prenatal care • Remote patient monitoring • Obstetrics • COVID-19

KEY POINTS

- Prenatal care can be provided through many modalities, including virtual care.
- Remote monitoring is a tool to use with virtual prenatal care visits and results in similar patient satisfaction as in-person care.
- When prenatal complications arise, the care team can transition back to in-person care. Better data and guidelines will be needed to improve the virtual management of pregnancy complications.
- Virtual care is growing as technology evolves for this population.

INTRODUCTION/BACKGROUND

The primary goal of prenatal care is the birth of a healthy infant while minimizing maternal morbidity and mortality. The current model of prenatal care for a low-risk pregnancy in the United States includes a recommended 12 to 14 in-person visits throughout a 40-week pregnancy, typically with visits every 4 weeks until 28 weeks, every 2 weeks until 36 weeks, and weekly thereafter.[1] Despite significant medical and technological advances, this schedule has remained largely unchanged since its inception in the early twentieth century, when it was developed primarily for the early detection of preeclampsia.[2] This coincided with physicians taking primary responsibility for prenatal care and the transition of more births to a hospital setting; before this development, prenatal care was provided primarily by nurses and community midwives, with births taking place primarily in the home.[2]

There are growing data to support fewer prenatal visits for low-risk pregnancies. A 2015 study examined two groups of patients: those with fewer than 10 prenatal visits and those with 10 or more prenatal visits. There was no difference in neonatal outcomes between the two groups, but patients with more visits were more likely to undergo induction of labor and had a higher rate of cesarean delivery.[3] Further, guidelines for prenatal care delivery vary significantly around the world. In a comparison of the United States to peer countries, there was little variation in prenatal care

Department of Family Medicine, Academic Office 112631 E 17th Ave, Aurora, CO 80045, USA
* Corresponding author.
E-mail address: Alison.Shmerling@cuanschutz.edu

Prim Care Clin Office Pract 49 (2022) 609–619
https://doi.org/10.1016/j.pop.2022.05.002
0095-4543/22/© 2022 Elsevier Inc. All rights reserved.

guidelines for educational topics and psychosocial services, but significant variation in visit frequency. Of eight peer countries, all but one recommended fewer visits throughout pregnancy. More than half recommended a total of 7 to 10 visits, and most recommended a longer interval between visits in the third trimester.[4]

There are ongoing efforts to optimize and enhance prenatal care, including the incorporation of telehealth modalities. Telehealth has been investigated both as an adjunct to routine care and the basis of a full redesign of the prenatal care paradigm. Telehealth has been well established in obstetric care to improve access to specialty care and ultrasound interpretation for patients in rural settings.[5] In some rural areas deemed maternity-care deserts due to lack of access to care, telemedicine has been used to supplement routine prenatal care and postpartum care.[5] Telemedicine has also been used to support rural providers. The University of Arkansas for Medical Sciences has implemented state-wide educational campaigns around hypertension and hemorrhage management for rural hospitals, as well as 24-h access to educational materials, a high-risk pregnancy call center, and maternal–fetal medicine consultation.[5] Text-message-based educational interventions have improved smoking cessation in pregnancy and breastfeeding rates at 6 months postpartum.[6] A telephone-based lifestyle intervention decreased weekly gestational weight gain in patients at risk for excessive gestational weight gain.[7] Smartphone applications for mood tracking have demonstrated improved identification and service delivery for patients with perinatal symptoms of depression.[8]

Other groups have studied reduced in-person care models supplemented with telehealth. In 2019, the Mayo Clinic published their work on the OB Nest model, which consists of eight in-person physician appointments, six virtual visits with a nurse, and access to an online community of other pregnant people. Patients were supplied with a home blood pressure (BP) cuff and fetal Doppler.[9] Compared with usual care, OB Nest patients had higher satisfaction, decreased pregnancy-related stress, and increased duration of breastfeeding, with no differences in perceived quality of care, adherence to the American College of Obstetricians and Gynecologists (ACOG) guidelines, and clinical maternal and fetal outcomes.[9] The study authors postulated that the increased satisfaction and decreased pregnancy-related stress could be due to receiving care from the comfort of home, access to an online community for support throughout pregnancy, and access to home monitoring devices for fetal heart rate and BP.[9] Another study assessed patient satisfaction with a hybrid model, in which prenatal patients during the COVID-19 pandemic had the option to receive routine care with 12 to 14 in-person visits, or with one-third of the visits as virtual visits. Both groups were highly satisfied with their care, but those who had opted for virtual care had significantly higher mean satisfaction scores.[10] This was thought to be due to a shared desire to limit in-person care during the pandemic.[10] An additional study assessed patient comfort with the use of technology and telemedicine for weekly blood glucose review, as opposed to in-person visits, in pregnancies complicated by gestational diabetes. Patients generally were satisfied with this care, believed it to be safe, and appreciated the convenience, but noted some discomfort with the use of the technology such as a home BP cuff and fetal Doppler.[11]

GUIDELINE SUMMARY

The American College of Obstetricians and Gynecologists[1]: ACOG recommends that obstetric visits be individualized (**Table 1**). They do recommend that women with known medical problems, complications with prior pregnancies, or those who had fertility treatment should be seen as early as possible. They acknowledge that

Table 1
Summary of national and international prenatal care guidelines

Organization	Initial Prenatal	Frequency of Visits	Total Visits
ACOG	Within the first trimester, and dating ultrasound ideally before 13 6/7 wk	Every 4 wk until 28 wk, every 2 wk until 36 wk, then weekly until delivery, but can be individualized	Individualized based on each patients' needs
AAFP	First trimester	No guideline	7–12 for developed countries
NICE	First trimester	See **Table 2**	10 for nulliparous patients and 7 for parous patients
WHO	Up to 12 wk	See **Box 1**	8 "contacts"

although a typical pregnant patient is seen every 4 weeks until 28 weeks, every 2 weeks until 36 weeks, then weekly after that, there are women that may need more or fewer visits depending on their circumstances.

The American Academy of Family Physicians (AAFP)[12]: The AAFP has no guidelines for the frequency of prenatal visits, but acknowledges that 7 to 12 visits are typical in developed countries.

The National Institute for Health and Care Excellence (NICE)[13]: NICE recommends 10 routine antenatal appointments with an OB provider for nulliparous women and 7 routine antenatal appointments with an OB provider for parous women. See the schedule timing in **Table 2**.

World Health Organization (WHO)[14]: The 2016 WHO Antenatal Care Model recommends a minimum of 8 antenatal care "contacts" during the pregnancy to reduce perinatal mortality and improve women's experience of care. See the schedule in **Table 2**. They prefer the word "contact" to "visit," as it implies an active connection between a pregnant woman and a health care provider that is not implicit with the word "visit." The term "contact" can be adapted to local contexts.

Evolution of Telehealth in Prenatal Care

The novel coronavirus disease 2019 (COVID-19) was first identified in Wuhan, China, in December 2019. By January 30, 2020, the WHO declared COVID-19 a public health emergency, and it was officially classified as a pandemic by the WHO on March 11, 2020.[15] This led to rapid changes in health care delivery throughout the world to limit viral exposure to patients and health care staff, as well as conservation of personal protective equipment. For some fields, this included canceling and postponing nonurgent care and procedures; for prenatal care, this led to creative reimaginings of care delivery and, in many cases, the incorporation of telehealth.

For the average low-risk pregnant patient, the goal at many institutions was to plan in-person visits around necessary in-person care and supplement with virtual visits.[16–19] This typically included in-person visits for:

- The initial maternity care intake for a dating ultrasound and prenatal laboratories
- 20 weeks for the anatomy ultrasound
- 28 weeks for glucose tolerance testing, repeat complete blood count (CBC), administration of the tetanus, diphtheria, and pertussis (TDaP) vaccine, and Rhogam administration if indicated

---

Box 1
2016 World Health Organization antenatal care model schedule

Contact 1: up to 12 wk

Contact 2: 20 wk

Contact 3: 26 wk

Contact 4: 30 wk

Contact 5: 34 wk

Contact 6: 36 wk

Contact 7: 38 wk

Contact 8: 40 wk

Adapted from World Health Organization. WHO recommendations on antenatal care for a positive pregnancy experience Updated 28 November 2016. Accessed December 1, 2021. https://www.who.int/publications/i/item/9789241549912.

- 36 weeks for a collection of the Group B streptococcal swab and determination of fetal presentation
- 39 weeks through delivery

Further modifications were required for high-risk pregnancies (eg, gestational diabetes, gestational hypertension, preeclampsia, and abnormal anatomy ultrasound) requiring closer monitoring, including pregnancies requiring more frequent ultrasounds, diagnostic procedures, and antenatal testing, which have limited options for conversion to telehealth.

Models of telehealth in prenatal care

Columbia University Irving Medical Center (CUIMC) in New York City examined the uptake of telehealth during the 5-week period from March 9 to April 12, 2020. Approximately, one-third of the 4248 total visits in the study period took place via telehealth, with an increase in the proportion each week to a peak of 50% to 60% of visits (via telehealth) by week 5, depending on the practice setting.[20] The CUIMC still attempted to

---

Table 2
National Institute for Health and Care Excellence Antenatal Care schedule

Appointments for All Pregnant Women	Additional Appointments for Nulliparous Women
Visit 1: First trimester	25, 31, and 40 wk
Ultrasound at 11 + 2–14 + 1 wk	
Visit 2: 16 wk (14–18 wk)	
Ultrasound at 18 + 0–20 + 6 wk	
Visit 3: 28 wk	
Visit 4: 34 wk	
Visit 5: 36 wk	
Visit 6: 38 wk	
Visit 7: 41 wk (for those that have not given birth)	

Data from National Institute for Health and Care Excellence. Antenatal care. Updated 19 August 2021. Accessed December 1, 2021. https://www.nice.org.uk/guidance/ng201/chapter/Recommendations.

limit exposure by clustering the scheduling of required in-person services to the same day.[21] They began recommending cell-free fetal DNA for aneuploidy screening to avoid multiple visits for blood draws and ultrasound for nuchal translucency.[21] They also published guidelines for modifications of virtual care models for high-risk pregnancies.[22] These guidelines included modified in-person visit schedules, recommendations for home equipment such as home BP monitoring, and modified antenatal testing schedules, depending on the high-risk feature. As an example, for hypertensive disorders of pregnancy, they recommend access to a home BP cuff for all patients and recommend in-person visits after 36 weeks gestation. Similar modifications are detailed for conditions including maternal cardiovascular disease, maternal neurologic conditions, gestational and non-gestational diabetes mellitus, history of preterm birth and stillbirth, fetal conditions such as intrauterine growth restriction (IUGR), multiple gestation, and congenital anomalies.[22] Providers surveyed during a 5 week period from March to April 2020 felt that telehealth increased access (97%), provided adequate care (92%, definition of "adequate care" not published), and that they would continue to use the technology after the pandemic (89%). Providers were divided on whether they felt there was any change in preparation time before the appointment (50%), documentation time (56%), and patient rapport (53%).[20]

The University of Michigan developed the "4-1-4 prenatal plan" which included four in-person visits (at 8 weeks, 28 weeks, 36 weeks, and 39 weeks), one antenatal ultrasound at 20 weeks, and four virtual visits (at <8 weeks for counseling, 16 weeks, 24 weeks, and 32 weeks).[17] They encouraged home monitoring of BP and fetal heart rate.[17] Patients were surveyed and a majority felt that the conversion to telehealth improved access to care (68.8%), believed the care to be safe (53.3%), and reported satisfaction with care (77.5%).[23] However, only 45.5% of patients felt that the quality of virtual care was the same as the quality of in-person care, and only 40.3% of patients reported willingness to continue with virtual visits after the pandemic.[23] Patients identified decreased provider continuity and relationship building as a driver behind these findings.[23] Providers felt that telehealth improved access (96.1%), believed the care to be safe (62.1%), and reported satisfaction (83.1%). In contrast to patients, 92.2% of providers reported a willingness to continue this care model after the pandemic.[23] Barriers that providers identified to successful prenatal telehealth care were difficulty with interpreter services, difficulties for patients accessing and using the technology, the additional training required for staff and physicians, as well as a concern that differential access to technology and the Internet may lead to inequitable access to care.[20,23]

Multiple studies demonstrated that the no-show rate did not increase after the transition to telehealth.[20,23] The Perinatal Experiences and COVID-19 Effects (PEACE) study also found that most of the women reported being very, extremely, or moderately satisfied (71.4%) with their virtual experiences, although 89.9% preferred in-person care in non-pandemic conditions. Satisfaction scores decreased with increased pandemic duration.[24] Given this discrepancy between patient and provider satisfaction, more research is needed to determine the drivers of these lower satisfaction scores. It will be important to continue to monitor patient satisfaction and experience to inform the future evolution of telehealth prenatal care.

Of note, utilization of telehealth for prenatal care and satisfaction of care via telehealth was not consistent across all patients. One study at NYU Langone Medical Center in New York City examined differential uptake of telehealth across demographics and found that patients with public insurance were less likely to have at least one telehealth visit when compared with patients with private insurance (60.9% vs 87.3%, P <.0001).[25] In addition, an inner-city safety-net hospital in New York City assessed patient satisfaction scores in patients who had at least one virtual visit and one in-person visit from March 2020 to May 2020. Although all scores were in the "satisfied" range, the satisfaction scores were lower in all categories for virtual visits.[26] Although telehealth has the potential to improve access to care in some settings, these data raise the concern that a transition to telehealth has the potential to deepen pre-existing disparities in prenatal and maternity care. More data are needed on the implementation of telehealth prenatal care in public insurance and safety-net populations to ensure appropriate care delivery.

EXAMPLE PRACTICES
Example Practice 1: UCHealth (University of Colorado) Family Medicine Residency Program, Denver, Colorado

AF Williams Family Medicine Center: mixed in-person and virtual visits
AF Williams Family Medicine Center introduced a schedule displayed in **Table 3**, composed of decreased in-person visits with a combination of virtual visits. For those patients with high-risk pregnancies, patients were only offered virtual visits with the approval of the provider. Each patient was given a home BP cuff for monitoring. In addition, patients were offered monthly group informative sessions via Zoom (Zoom Video Communications, Inc, San Jose, CA) based on trimester. These sessions were helpful to patients but not well attended (around 25%–50% attendance) and eventually ceased after 4 months. Over time, pregnant patients preferred to be seen in-person over virtual visits, and the clinic eventually stopped scheduling regular virtual visits once in-person visits increased. AF Williams still has virtual visits available

Table 3		
AF Williams Family Medicine Center schedule		
Maternity Care Visits	**Telehealth**	**In-Person**
New maternity care intake with nurse	X	
New maternity care intake with provider		X
16 wk		X
20 wk		Ultrasound visit
24 wk	X (at patient discretion)	
28 wk		X
32 wk		X
34 wk (with BP cuff)	X (at patient discretion)	
36 wk		X
37 wk (with BP cuff)	X at patient discretion))	
38 wk (with BP cuff)	X (at patient discretion)	
39 wk		X
40 wk		X
41 wk		X
Postpartum visit with baby (if the baby is AFW patient)		
2–3 d		X
2 wk		X
2 mo		X
Postpartum visit with no baby at AF Williams Family Medicine Center (AFW)		
2 wk and 6 wk	X	

to pregnant patients if they have issues with scheduling or coming to the clinic, but these visits have become rare.

Example Practice 2: UCHealth Family Medicine Practice Located in the Denver, Colorado Metropolitan Area

Westminster Family Medicine: virtual group prenatal care

To decrease the loneliness and isolation many pregnant women were experiencing during the pandemic for fear of contracting COVID while pregnant, UCHealth Westminster Family Medicine began virtual group prenatal visits (**Table 4**). The format consisted of six sessions, meeting once per month, which repeated continuously starting in January 2021. Patients started at any point in the curriculum, creating a group spanning all gestational ages. The project received funding from a Colorado Medicaid Upper Payment Limit Grant and purchased home Doppler monitors and BP cuffs for patients to use. Once monthly, a 2-hour block was used on the provider's schedule to see each of up to six patients in 10-min individual appointments, with a 1-hour talk from an external speaker and questions answered as a group. For most of the first year, the patients and speakers all met via Zoom. During the brief individual check-in, the provider was able to have the patient use the Doppler to auscultate fetal heart tones and check BP. Any upcoming laboratories were coordinated with the supporting medical assistant/project manager before or after the provider saw the patient. Patients were generally seen in person at least once per month, so patients occasionally end up having slightly more appointments in the first half of pregnancy. Ten prenatal patients participated in the program between January 2021 and October 2021. One notable complication arose where, due to inability to measure fundal heights, a patient had a presumed delay in diagnosis of sizes less than dates and subsequent concern for IUGR. Despite this concern, the baby was appropriate for gestational age at birth. Of note, the evidence to support the routine use of fundal height measurements as a screening tool to identify IUGR is inconclusive, although commonly still practiced as the standard of care.[27]

After the COVID-19 vaccine became available to patients, they were given the option to attend class in person, which after September 2021 all patients chose to do. The class is ongoing and maintains social distancing and masking in a large conference room with speakers still on Zoom. The curriculum topics (and presenter types) include peripartum mood changes (psychologist); normal vaginal delivery/non-pharmacologic pain management (doula); pharmacologic pain management (anesthesiologist); complications of pregnancy (maternal–fetal medicine provider [MFM]); C-sections, assisted delivery, the COVID vaccine in pregnancy (MFM); and breastfeeding (lactation consultant).

Example Practice 3: Web Application

Babyscripts[28] is an application that allows maternity providers to enroll their patients. The cost is several hundred dollars per patient. The patient receives a Bluetooth scale and BP monitor which synchronizes with the application. The patient checks in weekly with the application to review topics about her current stage of pregnancy, weigh herself, and check her BP. In addition, patients attend in-person appointments every 8 weeks until 32 weeks, then at 34, 36, 37, 38, and 39 weeks. In a study of 88 women, 47 were assigned to the "Babyscripts" group and 41 to the control group (standard care). Patients were allocated via quasi-randomization based on whether they had an iPhone. Although not powered to detect a difference in perinatal outcomes, the study showed a reduction in in-person visits in the Babyscripts group compared with the control group, and no statistically significant difference between patient or provider satisfaction.[29]

Table 4
Westminster Family Medicine: Proposed telehealth hybrid prenatal care schedule[a]

	First Trimester	Second Trimester				Third Trimester								
Weeks' Gestation	8	12	16	20	24	28	30	32	34	36	37	38	39	40
Required testing?	Laboratories, Pap	U/S		U/S		Glucose tolerance test (GTT), TDaP				Group B Strep (GBS) and confirm vertex				
Telehealth possible?	N	Y	Y	Y	Y	N	Y[a]	Y[a]	Y[a]	N	Y[a]	Y[a]	Y[a]	Y[a]

[a] Table assuming appropriate capacity for remote monitoring with blood pressure cuff and home Doppler and following WHO guidelines to include a minimum of 8 touchpoints during pregnancy, supplement per provider, and patient comfort. For complications of pregnancy, individual assessments based on the severity of complications need to be considered.

DISCUSSION

Using telehealth for prenatal care is still an evolving field, in which the COVID-19 pandemic has accelerated its use. There remain discussions on the appropriate number of prenatal visits for low-risk patients, with some evidence that not only does patient and provider satisfaction improve, fewer visits may also improve maternal outcomes such as fewer inductions of labor and cesarean sections without any differences in neonatal outcomes.

Virtual visits can be a valuable tool to improve access to prenatal care, especially in cases where clinics may limit in-person visits because of safety concerns or in more remote rural settings where access to maternity providers may be limited. Developing a hybrid model of care which includes a mix of in-person and virtual visits to include group visits can be an effective way to provide prenatal care and education. In low-risk pregnancies, as few as four in-person visits can be accomplished with the rest of the visits conducted virtually with remote BP and fetal heart tone monitoring. However, the most effective process to develop this workflow is still not clear. Prenatal patients have expressed satisfaction with virtual prenatal care, especially to limit in-person care to limit infection risk during the pandemic. However, when there were opportunities to be seen in person, especially as the COVID pandemic continued and in-person care returned, many patients choose to be seen in person.

Many questions remain with virtual prenatal care. There is no clear guidance on how to address pregnancy complications, which will usually result in converting virtual visits to in-person assessments. Concerns still exist on missing important complications that in-person visits may catch compared with virtual visits, such as growth restrictions, gestational hypertension, or preeclampsia. There is limited evidence on how to best use home monitoring such as blood pressure (BP) cuffs and fetal Doppler monitoring. Many barriers to this aspect of virtual care remain. Patients who received access to home fetal Dopplers may potentially have higher satisfaction with virtual care, but it is not known the true effect of home monitoring on satisfaction or outcomes. Lack of access to the technology to complete virtual visits, including home monitoring, may limit the effectiveness of virtual visits and widen health care disparities between patients. Other routine care such as assessing fetal growth with fundal heights is another challenge that may need more evidence to determine the appropriate frequency and accuracy of fundal heights, especially in later gestation.

Last, as we view virtual prenatal care as a way to improve access to care, caution is needed to assure virtual care does not cause a greater gap in health care disparities. Access to the technology required for successful virtual visits, such as appropriate Internet bandwidth, may be more available for some patients and less available to others. In addition, access to and comfort with the use of remote monitoring equipment is another factor that could add to health care disparities.

CLINICS CARE POINTS

Telehealth for prenatal care has shown significant promise. We make the following recommendations:

- For patients with low-risk pregnancies, we recommend following the World Health Organization guidelines to include a minimum of 8 touchpoints during pregnancy, with additional touchpoints based on provider and patient comfort (see **Table 4**).
- After 24 to 28 weeks, home Doppler and home blood pressure cuffs can support a more robust virtual care model.

- Patients need more education regarding when an in-person visit might be more appropriate if they choose to do more visits virtually. This can be done via an registered nurse (RN) educator, medical assistant (MA) educator, or prenatal education class model.
- Consider the impact of your virtual care model on disparities. For large volume practices, we recommend a quality improvement infrastructure during implementation to ensure you are not exacerbating existing disparities.

DISCLOSURE

None of the authors report any disclosures.

REFERENCES

1. American Academy of Pediatrics, American College of Obstetricians and Gynecologists. Guidelines for perinatal care. 8th edition. American Academy of Pediatrics; The American College of Obstetricians and Gynecologists; 2017. p. 691, xv.
2. Maloni JA, Cheng CY, Liebl CP, et al. Transforming prenatal care: reflections on the past and present with implications for the future. J Obstet Gynecol Neonatal Nurs 1996;25(1):17–23.
3. Carter EB, Tuuli MG, Caughey AB, et al. Number of prenatal visits and pregnancy outcomes in low-risk women. J Perinatol 2016;36(3):178–81.
4. Friedman Peahl A, Heisler M, Essenmacher LK, et al. A comparison of international prenatal care guidelines for low-risk women to inform high-value care. Am J Obstet Gynecol 2020;222(5):505–7.
5. Whittington JR, Ramseyer AM, Taylor CB. Telemedicine in Low-Risk Obstetrics. Obstet Gynecol Clin North Am 2020;47(2):241–7.
6. DeNicola N, Grossman D, Marko K, et al. Telehealth Interventions to Improve Obstetric and Gynecologic Health Outcomes: A Systematic Review. Obstet Gynecol 2020;135(2):371–82.
7. Ferrara A, Hedderson MM, Brown SD, et al. A telehealth lifestyle intervention to reduce excess gestational weight gain in pregnant women with overweight or obesity (GLOW): a randomised, parallel-group, controlled trial. Lancet Diabetes Endocrinol 2020;8(6):490–500.
8. Hantsoo L, Criniti S, Khan A, et al. A Mobile Application for Monitoring and Management of Depressed Mood in a Vulnerable Pregnant Population. Psychiatr Serv 2018;69(1):104–7.
9. Butler Tobah YS, LeBlanc A, Branda ME, et al. Randomized comparison of a reduced-visit prenatal care model enhanced with remote monitoring. Am J Obstet Gynecol 2019;221(6):638.e1-8.
10. Pflugeisen BM, Mou J. Patient Satisfaction with Virtual Obstetric Care. Matern Child Health J 2017;21(7):1544–51.
11. Harrison TN, Sacks DA, Parry C, et al. Acceptability of Virtual Prenatal Visits for Women with Gestational Diabetes. Womens Health Issues 2017;27(3):351–5.
12. Zolotor AJ, Carlough MC. Update on prenatal care. Am Fam Physician 2014; 89(3):199–208.
13. National Institute for Health and Care Excellence. Antenatal care. Updated 19 August 2021. Available at: https://www.nice.org.uk/guidance/ng201/chapter/Recommendations. Accessed December 1, 2021.

14. World Health Organization. WHO recommendations on antenatal care for a positive pregnancy experience Updated 28 November 2016. Available at: https://www.who.int/publications/i/item/9789241549912. Accessed December 1, 2021.
15. World Health Organization. Listings of WHO's response to COVID-19. Updated 29 June 2020. Available at: https://www.who.int/news/item/29-06-2020-covid timeline. Accessed November 15, 2021.
16. Fryer K, Delgado A, Foti T, et al. Implementation of Obstetric Telehealth During COVID-19 and Beyond. Matern Child Health J 2020;24(9):1104–10.
17. Peahl AF, Smith RD, Moniz MH. Prenatal care redesign: creating flexible maternity care models through virtual care. Am J Obstet Gynecol 2020;223(3):389.e1-10.
18. Zork NM, Aubey J, Yates H. Conversion and optimization of telehealth in obstetric care during the COVID-19 pandemic. Semin Perinatol 2020;44(6):151300.
19. Turrentine M, Ramirez M, Monga M, et al. Rapid Deployment of a Drive-Through Prenatal Care Model in Response to the Coronavirus Disease 2019 (COVID-19) Pandemic. Obstet Gynecol 2020;136(1):29–32.
20. Madden N, Emeruwa UN, Friedman AM, et al. Telehealth Uptake into Prenatal Care and Provider Attitudes during the COVID-19 Pandemic in New York City: A Quantitative and Qualitative Analysis. Am J Perinatol 2020;37(10):1005–14.
21. Aziz A, Fuchs K, Nhan-Chang CL, et al. Adaptation of prenatal care and ultrasound. Semin Perinatol 2020;44(7):151278.
22. Aziz A, Zork N, Aubey JJ, et al. Telehealth for High-Risk Pregnancies in the Setting of the COVID-19 Pandemic. Am J Perinatol 2020;37(8):800–8.
23. Peahl AF, Powell A, Berlin H, et al. Patient and provider perspectives of a new prenatal care model introduced in response to the coronavirus disease 2019 pandemic. Am J Obstet Gynecol 2021;224(4):384.e1-11.
24. Liu CH, Goyal D, Mittal L, et al. Patient Satisfaction with Virtual-Based Prenatal Care: Implications after the COVID-19 Pandemic. Matern Child Health J 2021;25(11):1735–43.
25. Limaye MA, Lantigua-Martinez M, Trostle ME, et al. Differential Uptake of Telehealth for Prenatal Care in a Large New York City Academic Obstetrical Practice during the COVID-19 Pandemic. Am J Perinatol 2021;38(3):304–6.
26. Futterman I, Rosenfeld E, Toaff M, et al. Addressing Disparities in Prenatal Care via Telehealth During COVID-19: Prenatal Satisfaction Survey in East Harlem. Am J Perinatol 2021;38(1):88–92.
27. Robert Peter J, Ho JJ, Valliapan J, et al. Symphysial fundal height (SFH) measurement in pregnancy for detecting abnormal fetal growth. Cochrane Database Syst Rev 2015;9:CD008136.
28. Babyscripts. Available at: Babyscripts.com. Accessed December 13, 2021.
29. Marko KI, Ganju N, Krapf JM, et al. A Mobile Prenatal Care App to Reduce In-Person Visits: Prospective Controlled Trial. JMIR Mhealth Uhealth 2019;7(5):e10520.

Telehealth and Hypertension Management

Robert J. Heizelman, MD

KEYWORDS

- Telehealth • Hypertension • Self-measurement of blood pressure
- Ambulatory blood pressure monitoring

KEY POINTS

- The COVID-19 pandemic has significantly accelerated telehealth.
- Hypertension can be accurately diagnosed by out-of-office blood pressure readings and treated via telehealth.
- Treatment of hypertension via telehealth is consistent with the concept of value-based care.

INTRODUCTION

Telehealth is recognized as one of the most rapidly growing areas in health care and is worthy of particular focus in today's health-care climate. Broadly considered, telehealth uses information and communication technologies to increase access and improve treatment in human health. These technologies have applications that are highly relevant to primary care, including home blood pressure (BP) monitoring. This article will examine the current state of telehealth concerning hypertension management.

Background

Hypertension is a leading cause of death and disability in the United States. It is second only to smoking as a preventable cause of death. Hypertension contributes to an increased risk of coronary heart disease, stroke, and end-stage renal disease.[1] Hypertension is a prevalent condition affecting approximately 45% of adults in the United States.[2]

In April 2021, the United States Preventive Services Task Force reaffirmed its 2015 recommendation for screening for hypertension in the adult population, based on a systematic review of literature after 2015.[3]

Department of Family Medicine, The University of Michigan, 300 North Ingalls Street, 4C06, Ann Arbor, MI 48109-5625, USA
E-mail address: roheizel@med.umich.edu

Prim Care Clin Office Pract 49 (2022) 621–629
https://doi.org/10.1016/j.pop.2022.05.003
0095-4543/22/© 2022 Elsevier Inc. All rights reserved.
primarycare.theclinics.com

In 2017, the American College of Cardiology/American Heart Association Task Force on Clinical Practice Guidelines attempted to answer 4 important questions related to the treatment of hypertension.[4]

1. Is there evidence that self-directed monitoring of BP and/or ambulatory BP monitoring are superior to office-based measurement of BP by a health-care worker for preventing adverse outcomes for which high BP is a risk factor and achieving better BP control?
2. What is the optimal target for BP lowering during antihypertensive therapy in adults?
3. In adults with hypertension, do various antihypertensive drug classes differ in their comparative benefits and harms?
4. In adults with hypertension, does initiating treatment with antihypertensive pharmacologic monotherapy versus initiating treatment with 2 drugs (including fixed-dose combination therapy), either of which may be followed by the addition of sequential drugs, differ in comparative benefits and/or harms on specific health outcomes?

The 2017 High Blood Pressure Clinical Practice Guidelines state "Out-of-office BP measurements are recommended to confirm the diagnosis of hypertension and for titration of BP-lowering medication, in conjunction with telehealth counseling or clinical interventions."[4] This is a Class of Recommendation (COR) of I, Level of Evidence (LOE) of A (Benefit>>>Risk, highest quality of evidence). The guidelines further recommend that patient training should occur under medical supervision, and that validated automated devices should be used, as well as a properly sized cuff.

BP readings can be broadly categorized as normal BP, elevated BP, stage 1 hypertension, and stage 2 hypertension. Treatment recommendations vary for these categories[4] (Fig. 1).

Normal BP is defined as less than 120/80 mm Hg. Patients with normal BP should be counseled regarding healthy lifestyles and reassessed annually.[4]

Elevated BP is defined as 120 to 129/<80 mm Hg. Patients with elevated BP should receive nonpharmacological treatment and be reassessed in 3 to 6 months.[4]

Stage 1 hypertension is defined as 130 to 139/80 to 89 mm Hg. Treatment depends on the presence or absence of atherosclerotic cardiovascular disease (ASCVD) or estimated risk of ASCVD greater than or equal to 10%. In the absence of ASCVD or risk factors, patient should receive nonpharmacological treatment and be reassessed in 3 to 6 months. In the presence of ASCVD or risk factors, patients should receive both non-pharmacological treatment and BP lowering medication and be reassessed in 1 month.[4]

Stage 2 hypertension is defined as greater than or equal to 140/90. Patients with stage II hypertension should receive both nonpharmacological treatment and BP lowering medication and be reassessed in 1 month.[4]

For initiation of treatment with antihypertensive medications, first-line agents include thiazide type diuretics, calcium channel blockers, and Angiotensin Converting Enzyme (ACE) inhibitors or Angiotensin Receptor Blocker (ARBs).[4]

Regarding choices for the initial monotherapy or combination therapy, recommendations vary depending on the classification of hypertension (stage 1 vs stage 2) and how far the patient is above the target BP. Initiation of treatment either with first-line agents or a combination agent is recommended for patients with stage 2 hypertension who are more than 20/10 mm Hg above the target BP. Initiation of treatment with a single agent is reasonable in patients with stage 2 hypertension.[4]

All patients with hypertension should initiate therapeutic lifestyle modifications including smoking cessation, control of blood sugar and blood lipid levels, dietary modifications (DASH), and physical activity.[5]

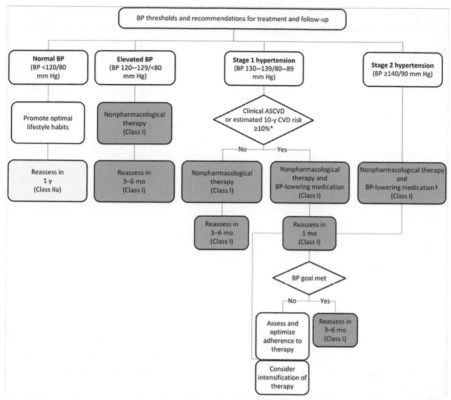

Fig. 1. BP thresholds and recommendations for treatment and follow-up. *Using the ACC/ AHA Pooled Cohort Equations. †Consider initiation of pharmacological therapy for stage 2 hypertension with 2 antihypertensive agents of different classes. (*From* Whelton PK, Carey RM, Aronow WS, et al. 2017 ACC/AHA/AAPA/ABC/ACPM/AGS/APhA/ASH/ASPC/NMA/PCNA Guideline for the Prevention, Detection, Evaluation, and Management of High Blood Pressure in Adults: Executive Summary: A Report of the American College of Cardiology/ American Heart Association Task Force on Clinical Practice Guidelines [published correction appears in Hypertension. 2018 Jun;71(6):e136-e139] [published correction appears in Hypertension. 2018 Sep;72(3):e33]. *Hypertension.* 2018;71(6):1269-1324.)

The importance of home BP monitoring cannot be overstated. Advantages of home BP monitoring include reproducibility and accuracy, the ability to aid in the detection of white coat hypertension and masked hypertension, and to aid in the risk stratification for cardiovascular disease and stroke (**Table 1**).[6]

DISCUSSION
Telehealth Techniques Improve Accuracy in Hypertension Diagnosis and Monitoring

The management of hypertension is complicated by the fact that in-office BP measurements may not accurately reflect the patient's BP. There are several classifications of hypertension including primary hypertension, secondary hypertension, masked hypertension, and white-coat hypertension. Masked hypertension is defined as normal BP readings in the office but elevated readings outside the clinical setting,

Table 1
Advantages and Limitations of Home Blood Pressure Monitoring

Advantages	Limitations
• Can take multiple readings during an extended period of time • Avoids white-coat reaction to BP measurement • Reproducible • Predicts CV morbidity and mortality better than office BP • Can diagnose white-coat and masked hypertension • Allows patients to better understand hypertension management • Telemonitoring allows remote monitoring by health-care professionals • Detects increased BP variability	• Some devices have been found to be inaccurate • Cuff placement can affect the accuracy • May induce anxiety and excessive monitoring • Risk of treatment change by patients based on casual home measurements without doctors' guidance • Lack of nocturnal recording • Not yet reimbursed by insurance companies in many countries

Abbreviations: BP, blood pressure; CV, cardiovascular.
Parati, G., Stergiou, G., Asmar, R. et al. European Society of Hypertension Practice Guidelines for home blood pressure monitoring. J Hum Hypertens 24, 779–785 (2010). https://doi.org/10.1038/jhh.2010.54.

which can occur in up to 10% of the population.[7] White-coat hypertension represents elevated BP readings in the office when actual hypertension does not exist, resulting in inaccurate diagnoses. The white-coat effect also results in elevated in-office BP readings in individuals who have been accurately diagnosed and are being treated for hypertension.[8]

Overall, in-office and out-of-office BP measurements vary with a certain degree of predictability. Clinic measurements are typically higher and home BP measurements correlate with daytime ambulatory BP measurements (**Table 2**).

Out-of-office measurements of BP more accurately reflect a patient's BP. These measurements include ambulatory blood pressure monitoring (ABPM) and self-measured blood pressure (SMBP). Ambulatory BP monitoring involves the patient

Table 2
Corresponding values of SBP/DBP for clinic, HBPM, daytime, nighttime, and 24-h ambulatory blood pressure monitoring

Clinic	HBPM	Daytime ABPM	Nighttime ABPM	24-h ABPM
120/80	120/80	120/80	100/65	115/75
130/80	130/80	130/80	110/65	125/75
140/90	135/85	135/85	120/70	130/80
160/100	145/90	145/90	140/85	145/90

Abbreviations: ABPM, ambulatory blood pressure monitoring; BP, blood pressure; DBP, diastolic blood pressure; HBPM, home blood pressure monitoring; SBP, systolic blood pressure.
From Whelton PK, Carey RM, Aronow WS, et al. 2017 ACC/AHA/AAPA/ABC/ACPM/AGS/APhA/ASH/ASPC/NMA/PCNA Guideline for the Prevention, Detection, Evaluation, and Management of High Blood Pressure in Adults: Executive Summary: A Report of the American College of Cardiology/American Heart Association Task Force on Clinical Practice Guidelines [published correction appears in Hypertension. 2018 Jun;71(6):e136-e139] [published correction appears in Hypertension. 2018 Sep;72(3):e33]. *Hypertension.* 2018;71(6):1269-1324.

using a device that measures BP at various intervals, typically every 15 to 30 minutes during the day and 30 to 60 minutes at night, for a 24-hour to 48-hour period. Data is then averaged and reported with daytime averages and nighttime averages. Limitations of ABPM include lack of availability to some patients and physicians and that a relatively finite amount of time is measured.[9,10]

Alternatively, self-measured BP is readily available and can measure BPs during a much longer period. SMBP is similar to office-based measurement with respect to technique. This includes cuff size selection and proper positioning, appropriate rest before reading, and avoiding medications and substances (eg, caffeine and nicotine) that can adversely affect the accuracy of the reading.[4] When measuring BP at home, the patient should remain still, sit correctly, take multiple readings, and record readings accurately. BPs should be taken in the seated position, upright with feet flat on the floor, and the BP cuff at the level of the heart. At least 2 readings, 1 minute apart, should be taken.[11] SMBP can be useful in the following situations: establishing a diagnosis of hypertension, monitoring the effects of medication changes, monitoring controlled hypertension, and confirming the diagnosis of resistant hypertension.

Interestingly, the Food and Drug Administration (FDA) does not require formal validation for a manufacturer to market a BP monitor. However, the American Medical Association (AMA) sponsors a website that has information about validated BP monitors. These monitors are validated for clinical accuracy through an independent review process known as validated device listing (VDL). Current information about approved devices can be found at https://www.validatebp.org/.

Home devices that currently meet the VDL Criteria are listed below by manufacturer and model (**Table 3**).

Telehealth Monitoring of Hypertension Improves Value Metrics (Patient Outcomes and Satisfaction Vis-à-vis Cost)

As health-care transitions from fee-for-service to fee-for-value, it will become increasingly important to determine the extent to which BP telemonitoring improves clinical outcomes, decreases cost, and improves patient-reported outcomes. A recent study found that BP telemonitoring is cost-effective and results in clinical benefits as well as patient-perceived value. Ionov and colleagues, assessed whether BP telemonitoring is conducive to a value-based approach, which includes clinical and economic effectiveness, and improvement in patient-reported outcome/experience measures.[12] They concluded that measurements of clinical benefit as well as patient-perceived value suggest that BP telemonitoring is cost-effective.

In patients treated for hypertension, home BP monitoring improves adherence to antihypertensive medication and long-term control rates.[13]

Similarly, the HOME BP (Home and Online Management and Evaluation of Blood Pressure) trial randomized patients to usual care (office visits) and self-monitoring of BP with guided management. This study concluded that "self-monitored BP led to better control of systolic BP after 1 year than usual care, with low incremental costs."[14] (**Fig. 2**)

Except for individuals aged more than 80 years, self-measurement of home BP resulted in better control of hypertension.

Telemonitoring of Hypertension Is System-Supported

Concerning quality measures, the Centers for Medicare & Medicaid Services (CMS) uses electronic clinical quality measures (eCQMs) in a variety of quality reporting and value-based purchasing programs. eCQMs are measures specified in a standard electronic format that use data electronically extracted from electronic health records

Table 3
Home blood pressure monitoring devices that currently meet the VDL criteria

Manufacturer	Model	Validation Protocols	Cuff Sizes (cm)
BodyTrace	BT105	ANSI/AAMI/ISO 81060–2:2013	Adult (22–32) Extended (22–42)
CareSimple	BT105	ANSI/AAMI/ISO 81060–2:2013	Adult (22–32) Extended (22–42)
Transtek	LS802-GS	ISO 81060–2:2018	Standard (22–32) Large (22–42) Extra Large (22–45)
Transtek	LS802-GP	ISO 81060–2:2018	Standard (22–32) Large (22–42) Extra Large (22–45)
Omron	HEM-9210T	ANSI/AAMI/ISO 81060–2:2009	Small (17–22) Wide Range (22–42) Extra Large (42–50)
Omron	HEM-920T	ANSI/AAMI/ISO 81060–2:2009	Adult (22–42)
Withings	WPM05	ANSI/AAMI/ISO 81060–2:2013	Integrated (22–42)
Microlife	BP3MX1-3C	BHS Revised Protocol: 1993	Small (14–22) Standard (22–32) Large (32–42)
Microlife	BP3MX1-3	BHS Revised Protocol: 1993	Small (14–22) Standard (22–32) Large (32–42)
Microlife	BP3MX1-4	BHS Revised Protocol: 1993	Small (14–22) Standard (22–32) Large (32–42)
Microlife	BP3MX1-1	BHS Revised Protocol: 1993	Small (14–22) Standard (22–32) Large (32–42)
Omron	BP7000	ANSI/AAMI/ISO 81060–2:2013	Adult (22–42)
Omron	BP7250	ANSI/AAMI/ISO 81060–2:2009	Adult (22–42)
Omron	BP7200	ANSI/AAMI/ISO 81060–2:2009	Adult (22–42)
Omron	BP7100	ANSI/AAMI/ISO 81060–2:2009	Adult (22–42)
Omron	BP5450	ANSI/AAMI/ISO 81060–2:2009	Adult (22–42)
Omron	BP5350	ANSI/AAMI/ISO 81060–2:2009	Adult (22–42)
Omron	BP7450	ANSI/AAMI/ISO 81060–2:2009	Adult (22–42)
Omron	BP7350	ANSI/AAMI/ISO 81060–2:2009	Adult (22–42)
Omron	BP5100	ANSI/AAMI/ISO 81060–2:2009	Adult (22–42)
Omron	BP5250	ANSI/AAMI/ISO 81060–2:2009	Adult (22–42)
Omron	BP7900	ANSI/AAMI/ISO 81060–2:2009	Adult (22–42)
A&D Medical	UA-1200BLE	ANSI/AAMI/ISO 81060–2:2009	Integrated (22–42)
Hillrom-Welch Allyn	H-BP100SBP	ANSI/AAMI/ISO 81060–2:2009	XS (15–24) Standard (22–42)
A&D Medical	UA-1030T	BHS Revised Protocol: 1993*	Small (16–24) Medium (23–37) Smooth Fit (23–37) Large (31–45)
A&D Medical	UA-705	BHS Revised Protocol: 1993*	Medium (23.8–36) Large (36–45)

* The British Hypertension Society protocol for the evaluation of blood pressure measuring devices.
Data from US Blood Pressure Validated Device Listing (VDL™). https://www.validatebp.org/. Accessed November 22, 2021.

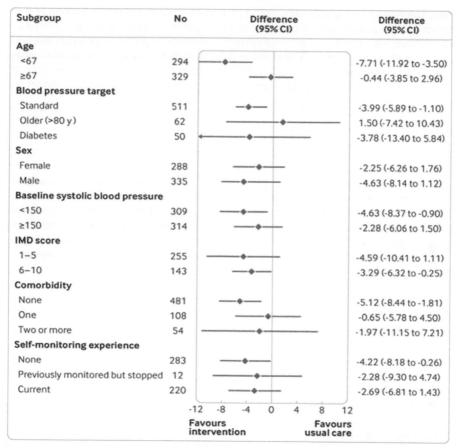

Fig. 2. Exploratory subgroup analyses showing effect sizes in usual care and intervention groups. (*From* McManus RJ, Little P, Stuart B, et al. Home and Online Management and Evaluation of Blood Pressure (HOME BP) using a digital intervention in poorly controlled hypertension: randomised controlled trial. BMJ. 2021;372:m4858. Published 2021 Jan 19.)

and/or health information technology systems to measure the quality of health care provided. eCQMs are assigned a Measure ID by CMS. Measure ID 165v10 pertains to hypertension management for the 2022 reporting year. The measure description is as follows: "Percentage of patients 18 to 85 years of age who had a diagnosis of essential hypertension starting before and continuing into, or starting during the first 6 months of the measurement period, and whose most recent blood pressure was adequately controlled (<140/90 mm Hg) during the measurement period." Starting in 2022, "blood pressure readings taken by a remote monitoring device and conveyed by the patient to the clinician are also acceptable." As home BP readings tend to be lower than in-office readings, this should result in a greater number of patients meeting the quality metric.[15]

The AMA previously developed and currently maintains current procedural terminology (CPT) codes. CPT codes exist for remote physiologic monitoring or RPM. Two codes pertain to SMBP: 99,473 and 99,474. CPT 99,473 is used for the initial setup of the equipment, patient education about the use of the equipment, and device calibration. CPT 99,474 is used for separate self-measurements of 2 readings 1 minute apart, twice daily during a 30-day period (minimum of 12 readings), collection of data reported by the patient and/or caregiver to the physician or other qualified health-care professional, with a report of average systolic and diastolic pressures and subsequent communication of a treatment plan to the patient. These codes can be used in asynchronous communication with the patient. The codes can be used alone or with a 25 modifier. This does not preclude evaluation and management coding (E&M) for telehealth.[16]

SUMMARY AND RECOMMENDATIONS

The 2017 Guideline for the Prevention, Detection, Evaluation, and Management of High Blood Pressure in Adults supports the practice with a Class of Recommendation (COR) of A and a LOE of I. Both (COR and LOE) are the highest possible. Self-measurement of BP is well supported by the research in its ability to improve measurement (and thus, diagnostic and treatment) accuracy, patient outcomes, as well as patient-perceived value. These objectives are achieved while retaining value and cost-effective service. Finally, procedures are in place to support implementation.

Home BP monitoring technologies will continue to evolve and patient interest in these technologies will likely increase. Health-care providers must consider using these technologies to provide better patient care. This recommendation is particularly relevant when considering the recent COVID-19 global pandemic and consequent recommendations for social distancing. SMBP will become increasingly important in assessing BP control through telehealth initiatives.

CLINICS CARE POINTS

- Out-of-office measurements of blood pressure (BP) more accurately reflect a patient's BP.
- BP targets and initial choice of medications are dependent on the stage of hypertension and comorbid conditions.
- For initiation of treatment with antihypertensive medications, first-line agents include thiazide type diuretics, calcium channel blockers, and ACE inhibitors or ARBs.

DISCLOSURE

The author is currently funded by the American Board of Family Medicine as a principal investigator for the evaluation of the Population Health Assessment Engine (PHATE).

REFERENCES

1. Virani SS, Alonso A, Benjamin EJ, et al. Heart disease and stroke statistics-2020 update: a report from the American heart association. Circulation 2020;141(9): e139–596.
2. Ostchega Y, Fryar C, Nwankwo T, et al. Hypertension prevalence among adults aged 18 and over: United States, 2017–2018. NCHS Data Brief 2020;364:1–8.
3. Guirguis-Blake JM, Evans CV, Webber EM, et al. Screening for hypertension in adults: updated evidence report and systematic review for the US Preventive services task force. JAMA 2021;325(16):1657–69.
4. Whelton PK, Carey RM, Aronow WS, et al. 2017 ACC/AHA/AAPA/ABC/ACPM/ AGS/APhA/ASH/ASPC/NMA/PCNA Guideline for the prevention, detection, evaluation, and management of high blood pressure in adults: a report of the

American college of cardiology/American heart association task force on clinical practice guidelines. Hypertension 2018;71(6):e13–115, published correction appears in Hypertension. 2018 Jun;71(6): e140-e144.

5. Williams B, Mancia G, Spiering W, et al, ESC Scientific document group. 2018 ESC/ESH guidelines for the management of arterial hypertension. Eur Heart J 2018;39(33):3021–104. Erratum in: Eur Heart J. 2019 Feb 1;40(5):475. PMID: 30165516.

6. George J, MacDonald T. Home blood pressure monitoring. Eur Cardiol 2015; 10(2):95–101.

7. Pickering TG, Eguchi K, Kario K. Masked hypertension: a review. Hypertens Res 2007;30(6):479–88.

8. Stergiou GS, Kario K, Kollias A, et al. Home blood pressure monitoring in the 21st century. J Clin Hypertens (Greenwich) 2018;20(7):1116–21.

9. Pickering TG, Miller NH, Ogedegbe G, et al. Call to action on use and reimbursement for home blood pressure monitoring: executive summary: a joint scientific statement from the American Heart Association, American Society of Hypertension, and Preventive Cardiovascular Nurses Association. Hypertension 2008; 52(1):1–9.

10. Pickering TG, White WB, American Society of Hypertension Writing Group. When and how to use self (home) and ambulatory blood pressure monitoring. J Am Soc Hypertens 2008;2(3):119–24.

11. Weinfeld JM, Hart KM, Vargas JD. Home blood pressure monitoring. Am Fam Physician 2021;104(3):237–43. PMID: 34523884.

12. Ionov MV, Zhukova OV, Yudina YS, et al. Value-based approach to blood pressure telemonitoring and remote counseling in hypertensive patients. Blood Press 2021;30(1):20–30. Epub 2020 Sep 21. PMID: 32954832.

13. Stergiou GS, Kollias A, Zeniodi M, et al. Home blood pressure monitoring: primary role in hypertension management. Curr Hypertens Rep 2014;16(8):462. PMID: 24924993.

14. McManus RJ, Little P, Stuart B, et al, HOME BP investigators. Home and online management and evaluation of blood pressure (HOME BP) using a digital intervention in poorly controlled hypertension: randomised controlled trial. BMJ 2021; 372:m4858. PMID: 33468518; PMCID: PMC7814507.

15. https://ecqi.healthit.gov/ecqm/ep/2022/cms165v10. Accessed June 2, 2022.

16. https://www.ama-assn.org/system/files/2020-06/smbp-cpt-coding.pdf. Accessed June 2, 2022.

Telehealth and Diabetes Management

Erik S. Kramer, DO, MPH, Dipl. of ABOM[a],*, Jill VanWyk, MD[a,b], Heather Holmstrom, MD[a,b]

KEYWORDS

• Virtual • Telehealth • Diabetes • Chronic care

KEY POINTS

• Diabetes is a chronic condition requiring frequent follow-up, which can be burdensome to patients.
• Virtual care is a useful tool as it can allow more rapid alterations in care plans.
• New technology can improve both patients' and providers' understanding of key elements of diabetes management.

BACKGROUND

Diabetes mellitus is a leading chronic disease worldwide, affecting more than 10% of adults in the United States. More than 33% of the United States population is at risk of prediabetes.[1] Among those at high risk and with impaired glucose, progression to type 2 diabetes can be significantly reduced with intensive lifestyle interventions, medication therapy, self-management, education, and clinical monitoring.[2] Diabetes can lead to systemic complications including neuropathy, retinopathy, nephropathy, coronary arterial disease, and stroke. The early morbidity and mortality and financial costs make this a critical public health condition.[2] Economic, regional, and social factors can influence access to regular diabetes care. The use of telehealth may help decrease the barriers to care, improve access, improve self-management, and decrease these long-term health care costs.

Approach to Virtual Care and the Patient with Diabetes

Patients with diabetes are commonly followed in the clinic every 3 to 6 months to provide a treatment and self-management plan, review bloodwork results, and complete a focused physical examination. With the advent and improvement of home monitoring devices and tools, most diabetes care can be completed virtually. The use of telehealth and eHealth tools can improve patient engagement and improve health

[a] University of Colorado, Anschutz; [b] UC Health Family Medicine - Boulder, 5495 Arapahoe Ave, Boulder, CO 80303, USA
* Corresponding author. 7403 Church Ranch Road #107, Westminster, CO 80021.
E-mail address: Erik.Kramer@cuanschutz.edu

Prim Care Clin Office Pract 49 (2022) 631–639
https://doi.org/10.1016/j.pop.2022.04.007
0095-4543/22/Published by Elsevier Inc.

primarycare.theclinics.com

Table 1
Recommended virtual schedule

Virtual Visit (Every 3–6 mo)	Laboratory Testing and Referrals	Patient at Home Resources
Assess glycemic control using at home A1c test and/or smart glucose self-monitoring, and assess for hypoglycemia	A1c: Every 3 mo if ≥ 8%, every 6 mo < 8% (depending on patient centered goal)	Blood Glucose Log (https://hopkinsdiabetesinfo.org/glucose-logs/)
Blood Pressure measured at home Assess Cholesterol medication adherence and the need for lipid testing	Cholesterol: Annually if above target. Consider every 3 y if on stable statin and/or LDL on target	AHA Blood Pressure Log (https://tinyurl.com/sre6nm7a) Recommended Blood Pressure Devices (https://www.validatebp.org)
Exercise, healthy eating, and weight check (at home scale)	eGFR, urine ACR: Annually	Exercise videos (www.diabetesstrong.com)
Self-screening for feet using at home Ipswich touch test[a]	Retinopathy screening: Annually	
Smoking cessation		
Self-management support (provide apps, support medication adherence, extend prescription refills until the next scheduled visit		Diabetes Foot Care (https://www.cdc.gov/diabetes/library/features/healthy-feet.html) Financial Relief and support (https://www.diabetes.org/resources/health-insurance)

[a] Ipswich Touch Test for evaluating the development of neuropathy involves having the patient lightly and briefly (1–2 s) touching the tips of the first, third, and fifth toes of both feet with the index finger to detect a loss in sensation (sensitivity 78.3%, specificity 93.9%).[22]

Adapted with permission from Kiran T, Moonen G, Bhattacharyya OK, et al. Managing type 2 diabetes in primary care during COVID-19. Can Fam Physician. 2020;66(10):745-747.

outcomes. Using telehealth in diabetes care may have a positive impact on diabetes outcomes including HbA1c levels. However, it is important to keep in mind technical barriers that may limit access for geriatric and underserved patients, and thus possibly worsen diabetes control.[3,4]

Completing a virtual visit may improve overall patient engagement. It may help patients engage with the clinical team through quicker medication adjustment, address urgent patient concerns before they become an emergency, and decrease the burden of access to transportation or leaving work that may result in no-shows for in-clinic visits. Virtual diabetes visits should be scheduled and completed based on the current standard of care. However, more frequent visits may be needed for those with more complicated issues.[5] **Table 1** provides a recommended schedule for diabetes care provided in a virtual format.

Evaluation of the Patient with Diabetes

Before the scheduled online visit, staff can contact patients to upload glucose meter data using the appropriate free and secure Internet platforms compatible with their devices and computer (**Table 2**). These platforms can be set up and accessed by clinical staff to review relevant data, including average daily glucose, average highs and lows, and overall blood glucose control within the recommended patient-centered goals.

The telehealth visit is conducted like an in-clinic office visit. **Box 1** provides examples of how to conduct a telehealth physical examination using video conferencing. The chief complaint, history of present illness (HPI), and review of systems (ROS) are easily obtainable via telehealth.[6] A focused review and update of the patient's medical/family/social history can be obtained, and medication review is often enhanced by the patient being at home and able to easily access their medications.[7] The first step when completing a comprehensive diabetes evaluation virtually is to review and assess the medical history, including any health changes as the prior encounter. A patient's risk for complications can be clarified by understanding the length of their illness as well as any comorbid conditions.

It is vital to complete a full review of a patient's current diabetes treatment plan, including current medications and glucose readings. Using an at-home A1c testing option, a patient's A1c can be completed before the visit to help support management changes and next steps. There are several brands for A1C testing kits such as Polymer Technology systems, CVS at home A1C test kits, and ReliOn fast A1C tests that are appropriate for home testing. Patients should be reminded that home A1c testing is not approved to diagnose diabetes. Alternatively, patients may be able to complete screening laboratories before the virtual visit.

The evaluation of diabetes should also include any episodes of hypoglycemia and how often and when they are occurring.

History of diabetes-related complications should be discussed and evaluated for new symptoms.

- Microvascular: Nephropathy (polyuria, urine output), retinopathy (blurry vision, visual disturbances), neuropathy (tingling, numbness, pain)
- Macrovascular: Cardiac (chest pain, palpitations, dyspnea on exertion, lower ext. swelling), peripheral arterial disease (claudication).
- Other: sexual dysfunction, gastroparesis.
- Assess additional risk factors for atherosclerosis: Tobacco use, obesity, family history

Diabetes self-management education and support can help facilitate the knowledge and skills to manage diabetes and improve self-care optimally. These should be assessed and incorporated into the virtual visit longitudinally.[8]

- Eating patterns and meal planning

Review individualized eating patterns and metabolic goals to determine the best eating pattern for the patient. Reducing overall carbohydrate intake has demonstrated the best evidence for improving hyperglycemia. The use of digital tools such as nutrition apps helps patients monitor their intake and make healthy diet choices acceptable for the management of diabetes.

Referral to a diabetic educator may be appropriate to support the patient's goals. If available, a virtual handoff with an in-clinic or system diabetic educator can help minimize access barriers.

- Weight management

A 5% to 7% weight reduction is recommended and often needed to help patients attain lipids, blood pressure, and glycemic goals.[9] While no single approach has been shown to be the best, a structured and individualized meal plan should be considered.

- Physical activity

Most adults with type 2 diabetes should engage in at least 150 minutes of moderate-intensity aerobic activity or 75 minutes of vigorous activity per week.[10]

All should decrease the amount of sedentary time and disrupt prolonged sitting. Many simple step counters or more advanced smartwatches/trackers can assist providers in understanding a patient's baseline level of activity so providers can tailor an exercise prescription to the specific needs of each individual.

- Psychosocial care

Psychosocial care should be integrated and patient-centered with collaboration with the local psychology team or embedded behavioral health in the patient's medical home.

Comprehensive assessment with screening focused on patient attitudes toward diabetes, expectations for medical management, and diabetes-related quality of life should be completed. Psychological and social problems can impair a patient's ability to self-manage diabetes. A multi-disciplinary team including a psychologist and social worker can be integrated virtually to help support a more comprehensive assessment and treatment plan.

Digital Tools for Self-Management and Education

When patients with diabetes have information and the necessary support to manage their diabetes, they often experience fewer subsequent diabetes-related complications and improved quality of life.[11] Participating in a self-management education program can help develop skills to manage diabetes which include checking blood sugars regularly, maintaining a diabetic-appropriate diet, maintaining an active lifestyle, and taking medications as prescribed. A number of self-management resources are available, with many at little to no cost to the patient (**Table 3**).

Table 2 Self management resources		
Tool		
Diabetes Self-Management Program (DSMP)	6 wk group program developed at Stanford University to help manage diabetes symptoms and help better manage diabetes day to day	https://www.selfmanagementresource.com/index.php/programs/small-group/diabetes-self-management/
Abacus Diabetes Care Rewards Program	provider-centric approach to care coordination by closing gaps in care	https://www.abacushealth.com/diabetes-program/
Better Choices, Better Health	Based on DSMP Stanford 6 wk program to empower self-management with digital tools, group support, and coaching	https://www.canaryhealth.com/bcbh-better-choices-better-health/
HabitNu DPP	In-person Medicare Diabetes Prevention Program – developed for both virtual and in-person delivery through weekly coaching and digital tools use.	https://habitnu.com/

Box 1
Example of telehealth physical examination using video conferencing

Step 1: Vital Signs	• Weight, blood pressure, pulse, oxygen saturation, temperature
Step 2: Skin assessment	• New bruises, rash, swelling
Step 3: Head, Eyes, Ears, Nose, and Throat	• Assess vision, observe conjunctiva, hearing, observe inside mouth and tongue
Step 4: Neck	• Assess pain with rotation, jugular venous distension
Step 5: Lungs	• Deeply inhale and hold; observe wheezing and tachypnea or labored breathing
Step 6: Heart	• Assess pulse; incorporate data from wearables
Step 7: Abdomen	• Assess if abdomen is firm, tender, or distended
Step 8: Extremities	• Press thumb into pre-tibial area and assess edema; perceived temperature observe feet for ulceration Complete Ipswich Touch Test
Step 9: Neurological	• Speech, gait, stand from seated position
	• Observe orientation and thought process

Adapted from Benziger CP, Huffman MD, Sweis RN, Stone NJ. The Telehealth Ten: A Guide for a Patient-Assisted Virtual Physical Examination. Am J Med. 2021 Jan;134(1):48-51.

Diet and physical activity

There are many digital apps now available to help patients monitor their food choices and caloric intake. Features include extensive food databases allowing patients to search nutritional information, including carbohydrates per serving, fiber content, and calories. Data can be shared with providers to help patients develop patient-centered goals and manage weight loss when appropriate (see **Table 3**).[12]

Self-monitoring of blood glucose

One of the most significant challenges seen in managing diabetes is controlling blood glucose adequately and consistently to prevent neuropathy, retinopathy, and

Table 3
Exercise, diet, and medication adherent apps

Exercise and Physical Activity	
My Fitness Pal	https://www.myfitnesspal.com
Nike Training	https://www.nike.com/ntc-app
Strava	https://www.strava.com
Diet	
CarbsControl	http://www.diabetesincontrol.com/carbscontrol-carb-tracker/
Lose It	https://www.loseit.com
Weight Watchers	https://www.weightwatchers.com/us/
Calorie King	https://www.calorieking.com/us/en/
Medication Adherence	
MedActionPlan	https://medactionplan.com/mymedschedule/
MyMeds	https://my-meds.com
Mydiabeteshome	MyDiabetesHome.com
RxmindMe Prescription	https://rxremindme.com
Glucometer Online Portals	
Freestyle Libre LibreView	https://provider.freestyle.abbott/
Dexcom Continuous Glucose Monitor	https://clarity.dexcom.com/professional/

nephropathy. Continuous glucose monitoring may improve overall control and reduce the risk of hypoglycemia. Fingerstick blood glucose tests are often used to monitor control; however, these provide data from only a single point in time. A1c testing shows the average daily blood sugar over the last 2 to 3 months but fails to inform patients and providers of daily glucose variability and time spent outside of the glucose target range.[13] Although self-monitoring blood glucose in noninsulin patients has not consistently shown significant improvements in A1c, it may be helpful when there is a change in management—diet, medications, physical activity.[14] Self-monitoring blood glucose in noninsulin type 2 diabetic patients should be implemented with training for both physicians and patients.[14] Patient training can be facilitated using a virtual visit with in-clinic nursing. Several blood glucose monitors have been developed to support this advanced monitoring.[15]

Contour next one smart meter and contour diabetes app (fingerstick)

- Integrates blood glucose meter with a smartphone app to manage blood glucose throughout the day

Dexcom G6 continuous glucose monitoring system

- Uses a small sensor under the skin and is connected to a smartphone app via a transmitter for continuous monitoring. Blood glucose can be shown as trends over time, increasing knowledge of whereby blood glucose is heading.

Fora TN'G voice blood glucose meter (fingerstick)

- Guides the user through testing and speaking out results—an option for the visually impaired.

Freestyle Libre continuous glucose monitoring

- Checks glucose without fingersticks through a reader or digital phone app. Can detect low or high glucose readings without scanning to notify patient to take immediate action.

Smart Meter's iGlucose diabetes management solution (fingerstick)

- Uses cellular-enabled solutions to automatically transmit real-time blood glucose results to health care professionals to make quick clinical decisions toward better blood glucose control.

Foot care

Diabetic foot care is an essential part of comprehensive diabetes care. Complications of poorly controlled diabetes include diabetic foot ulcers resulting in infections and amputation. Diabetes remains the most common cause of nontraumatic limb amputation.[16]

Both self-care to prevent ulcers and remote monitoring for established diabetic ulcers has advanced, and several medical devices are available.[16,17]

- The Podimetrics Mat is a "smart bathmat" that can mitigate complications by identifying foot ulcers early at home.[18] It captures foot temperatures and tracks the risk for ulceration.[19]
- The Orpyx's SurroSense Rx was developed to be used as an insole that can track and manage diabetic peripheral neuropathy-related complications.[20] Through a wearable smartwatch, plantar pressures are tracked, and users are alerted if pressures are above a threshold for a prolonged period of time. These data

can be easily shared with one's health care provider. Users can take action to minimize the risk of pressure-related ulcers forming.

The Ipswich touch test is a simple method for patients can assess their own risk for foot ulceration. The touch test has been found to have similar sensitivities and specificities as in-office monofilament testing. The Ipswich test involves lightly touching the tip of an index finger for 1 to 2 secs on the tips of the first, third, and fifth toes and the dorsum of the hallux of both feet.[21]

SUMMARY

Virtual care of patients with diabetes brings both challenges and opportunities. Patients may have easier access to health care by removing barriers such as transportation. They may more easily be able to describe how medications are taken and describe daily habits. Challenges arise in obtaining reliable information about glycemic control, blood pressure, and skin sensation and integrity.

Clinicians who wish to provide excellent telehealth care for patients should be aware of the technology available. Home A1C testing, as well as shared data from glucometer readings, can guide adjustments in medications. Patients may also wish to have laboratory work conducted before an appointment at a more convenient time for them or their caregivers. Patients can also be instructed in physical examination techniques to obtain further information about volume status and sensation.

Diabetic education and nutrition support as well as behavioral health support can be delivered via telehealth as well. Patients may be able to participate in nutrition education from their own kitchens providing opportunities for new ways to integrate health information. Lifestyle change support can also be accessed through digital technology. Multiple nutrition apps are available which allow for monitoring and education to support weight loss. Advanced technology to support the early detection of skin breakdown is available for selected patients at risk of foot ulcer.

CLINICS CARE POINTS

- Diabetes Mellitus is a chronic condition requiring frequent follow-up and monitoring.
- Telehealth offers unique opportunities to support our patients.
- A thorough diabetes-focused history allows the clinician to address patient concerns regarding diabetic care as well as Identify potential problems.
- Multiple technologies exist to help support glycemic control such as smart glucometers and home A1C tests.
- Laboratory examinations can be obtained at patient's convenience outside of restraints of provider's schedules.
- Ancillary support such as diabetic education, behavioral health support, and nutrition counseling can be delivered virtually.
- Clinicians should be aware of the technology available to support patient's lifestyle goals and provide early detection for diabetic-specific complications.

DISCLOSURE

There are no financial conflicts of interest to disclose.

REFERENCES

1. Centers for Disease Control and Prevention. National diabetes statistics report. 2020. Available at. https://www.cdc.gov/diabetes/pdfs/data/statistics/national-diabetes-statistics-report.pdf. Accessed October 10, 2021.
2. Forouhi NG, Wareham NJ. Epidemiology of diabetes. Medicine (Abingdon) 2014; 42(12):698–702.
3. Finkelstein J, Knight A, Marinopoulos S, et al. Enabling patient-centered care through health information technology. Evid Rep Technol Assess (Full Rep) 2012;(206):1–1531.
4. Jimison H, Gorman P, Woods S, et al. Barriers and drivers of health information technology use for the elderly, chronically ill, and underserved. Evid Rep Technol Assess (Full Rep 2008;175:1–1422.
5. Kiran T, Moonen G, Bhattacharyya OK, et al. Managing type 2 diabetes in primary care during COVID-19. Can Fam Physician 2020;66(10):745–7.
6. What is chief complaint and history of present illness. 2012. Available at. https://whatismedicalinsurancebilling.org/2012/09/what-is-chief-complaint-and-history-of.html. Accessed December 13, 2021.
7. Calloway S, Guenther J, Merrill E. 5-step guide for performing physical exams via telehealth. Available at. https://www.clinicaladvisor.com/home/topics/practice-management-information-center/5-step-guide-physical-exam-via-telehealth/. Accessed December 13, 2021.
8. American Diabetes Association. 5. Facilitating behavior change and well-being to improve health outcomes: <em>standards of medical care in diabetes—2021</em&gt. Diabetes Care 2021;44(Supplement 1):S53.
9. American Diabetes Association. 8. Obesity management for the treatment of type 2 diabetes: standards of medical care in diabetes-2021. Diabetes Care 2021; 44(Suppl 1):S100–10.
10. Janssen Pharmaceuticals Inc. Diabetes care primer for case managers. a guide for managing patients With type 2 diabetes. 2021. Available at. https://www.carepathhealthyengagements.com/sites/carepathhealthyengagements.com/files/T2D-case-manager-primer.pdf. Accessed December 13.
11. Centers for Disease Control and Prevention. National center for chronic disease prevention and health promotion division of population health. Managing Diabetes 2018. Available at. https://www.cdc.gov/learnmorefeelbetter/programs/diabetes.htm. Accessed December 13, 2021.
12. Shah VN, Garg SK. Managing diabetes in the digital age. Clin Diabetes Endocrinol 2015;1:16. https://doi.org/10.1186/s40842-015-0016-2.
13. Shrivastav M, Gibson W Jr, Shrivastav R, et al. Type 2 diabetes management in primary care: the role of retrospective, professional continuous glucose monitoring. Diabetes Spectr 2018;31(3):279–87. https://doi.org/10.2337/ds17-0024.
14. Polonsky WH, Fisher L. Self-monitoring of blood glucose in noninsulin-using type 2 diabetic patients: right answer, but wrong question: self-monitoring of blood glucose can be clinically valuable for noninsulin users. Diabetes Care 2012; 36(1):179–82.
15. American Diabetes Association. 7. Diabetes technology: <em>standards of medical care in diabetes—2021</em&gt. Diabetes Care 2021;44(Supplement 1):S85.
16. Armstrong DG, Boulton AJM, Bus SA. Diabetic foot ulcers and their recurrence. N Engl J Med 2017;376(24):2367–75.

17. Basatneh R, Najafi B, Armstrong DG. Health sensors, smart home devices, and the internet of medical things: an opportunity for dramatic improvement in care for the lower extremity complications of diabetes. J Diabetes Sci Technol 2018; 12(3):577–86.
18. Podimetrics podimetrics smartmat. Available at. https://www.podimetrics.com. Accessed December 13, 2021.
19. Frykberg RG, Gordon IL, Reyzelman AM, et al. Feasibility and efficacy of a smart mat technology to predict development of diabetic plantar ulcers. Diabetes Care 2017;40(7):973–80.
20. Orpyx SI. Sensory insoles. Available at. http://orpyx.com. Accessed December 13, 2021.
21. Rayman G, Vas PR, Baker N, et al. The ipswich touch test: a simple and novel method to identify inpatients with diabetes at risk of foot ulceration. Diabetes Care 2011;34(7):1517–8.
22. Sharma S, Kerry C, Atkins H, et al. The ipswich touch test: a simple and novel method to screen patients with diabetes at home for increased risk of foot ulceration. Diabet Med 2014;31(9):1100–3.

Virtual Care for Behavioral Health Conditions

Christina S. Palmer, MD[a],*, Shandra M. Brown Levey, PhD[a], Marisa Kostiuk, PhD[b], Aimee R. Zisner, PhD, MSc[a], Lauren Woodward Tolle, PhD[a], Rebecca M. Richey, PsyD[b], Stephanie Callan, MA[c]

KEYWORDS

- COVID-19 • Telehealth • Behavioral health

KEY POINTS

- The COVID-19 pandemic continues to highlight the immense need for more behavioral health care services, particularly services embedded in the primary care setting whereby many patients present first and solely for their mental health needs.
- Virtual care provides opportunities for prompt and improved access to behavioral health services.
- Virtual behavioral health is helping to support reducing health care disparities, particularly among rural and at-risk populations.

INTRODUCTION

The COVID-19 pandemic has highlighted the urgent need for behavioral health care services.[1] At the same time, the pandemic thrust virtual care forward out of necessity. A substantial portion of mental health care transitioned to virtual care during the COVID-19 pandemic, remains virtual today, and may persist in the future.

Mental health conditions are very common affecting about 20% of adults.[2] They include a wide array of disorders that cause changes in emotion or behavior, and these can cause problems with the quality of life, relationships, and school or job function. There are many challenges and barriers to high-quality and accessible mental health care, and primary care providers (PCPs) often take on the management of mental health conditions.[3]

Before the COVID-19 pandemic, there were known benefits to virtual behavioral health. Studies had shown that it was effective for managing and treating mental health conditions, with similar or better outcomes compared with in-person care. Studies had also demonstrated that telehealth could increase access for people,

[a] Department of Family Medicine, University of Colorado School of Medicine; [b] University of Colorado; [c] University of Colorado Denver
* Corresponding author.
E-mail address: Christina.Palmer@cuanschutz.edu

Prim Care Clin Office Pract 49 (2022) 641–657
https://doi.org/10.1016/j.pop.2022.04.008
0095-4543/22/© 2022 Elsevier Inc. All rights reserved.

particularly in rural locations. Importantly, patients were satisfied with virtual health and were found to still be able to create a therapeutic relationship with their provider.[4]

Yet, telehealth for mental health had not seen significant uptake, until the rapid shift to virtual care with the COVID-19 pandemic.[5] Virtual visits for behavioral health increased significantly, while there was also an increased need for behavioral health care.[6] Data around the benefits of telehealth for mental health at the system, provider, and patient level became clear. There were also evident barriers and challenges to virtual behavioral health care, highlighting areas to research and continue to improve.

As mental health needs continue to increase, access to timely evaluation from mental health providers decreases, and PCPs manage more complex behavioral health needs, there is an opportunity for the growth of effective, accessible, and affordable virtual integration of behavioral health services. In addition, payors are increasingly providing telehealth coverage for mental health services making it an option for more people. Here, we review the current state and future directions of behavioral health care via telehealth.

State of Virtual Behavioral Health Before COVID-19

Synchronous virtual delivery of behavioral health care was a rarity before the COVID-19 pandemic. Despite providing time savings, increased patient access, high user satisfaction, and comparable therapeutic alliance and clinical effectiveness to face-to-face visits across varied clinical populations and psychotherapies,[7,8] just 7% of prepandemic clinical work performed by psychologists was virtual.[9]

Factors accounting for this slow rate of adoption can be distilled into 3 domains including provider factors, patient factors, and policy/reimbursement barriers. In a pre–COVID-19 study of 1400 US-based psychologists, the most frequently cited deterrents to virtual behavioral health use were insufficient proficiency or knowledge to use virtual behavioral health in their practice (28.4% of respondents), client safety/crisis concerns (28%), privacy/HIPAA concerns (27%), and legality/interjurisdictional practice concerns (25.1%).[10]

From the patient perspective, barriers to virtual behavioral health include those related to access issues (eg, need for reliable Internet, phones with cameras and data, private spaces) and difficulties using virtual technologies (eg, among older adults and individuals with certain disabilities, such as those with visual, hearing, or severe attentional difficulties) as well as concerns surrounding trust, privacy, and security.[11,12] Importantly, many of these patient-related barriers remain, particularly among those that are underserved,[13] despite burgeoning acceptance of virtual behavioral health by providers, organizations, and the psychotherapy-seeking population as a whole.

Finally, policy and reimbursement barriers precluded widespread adoption of virtual behavioral health before the COVID-19 pandemic. Such barriers included restrictions based on geographic location, mode of delivery of services (eg, telephone vs video), and licensure qualifications of behavioral health providers. However, even before COVID-19, some advances expanded coverage and reimbursement for virtual behavioral health. For example, a 2018 federal ruling allowed veterans to access telehealth services including behavioral health visits, across states.[14] Before COVID-19, Medicare coverage of virtual behavioral health visits was permitted but was limited to patients residing in designated rural areas and visits conducted from an approved originating site, such as a clinic, hospital, or certain medical facilities.[15] Availability of virtual behavioral health services for patients with Medicare was expanded in 2019 to the treatment of substance use disorders and cooccurring mental illnesses regardless of the rural status of the patient.[16]

Although individual states and health insurances continue to differ in terms of their coverage for virtual behavioral health services,[17] the COVID-19 pandemic ushered in a new era of virtual behavioral health associated with expanded access and increased acceptance by patients, providers, and organizations.

Efficacy of Virtual Mental Health Services

While not a new method of delivering behavioral health care, virtual mental health service delivery was not widely used, and certainly not at the rate it has been used currently, before the COVID-19 pandemic. One reason for this has been provider preference or the belief that in-person behavioral health care is superior in quality and achieving improvements in functioning or reduction in symptomatology.

Multiple systematic reviews have examined the literature to determine if this belief is supported by research. In 2013, Hilty and colleagues[4] reviewed 70 studies researching the effectiveness of interventions comparing telehealth and in-person care. Findings from this review support telehealth as effective for multiple populations (eg, geriatric, adult, pediatric, underserved, rural, and ethnically diverse) in producing the same outcomes as in-person care (eg, reduction in depression, panic symptoms, reduced hospitalization, improved adherence, high satisfaction).

In some cases, telehealth was reported as superior to in-person care in its ability to allow for non-English speaking patients to connect with off-site bilingual providers as well as its acceptability in primary care settings for the collaboration of care.[4] Additional systematic reviews and meta-analyses have reported that telehealth yields comparable results to in-person care for the treatment of depression and anxiety and posttraumatic stress disorder (PTSD), particularly when cognitive behavioral therapy is used.[4,18,19] Randomized controlled trials have also found telehealth to be as effective as in-person behavioral health care for the treatment of PTSD,[20] bulimia,[21] and even anger management.[22]

Additional concerns that have potentially hindered the uptake of telehealth for behavioral health treatment are beliefs that telehealth negatively impacts the therapeutic alliance or the degree to which clinicians can effectively build rapport with their patients, and that patients would not want to engage in this type of treatment. Concerns have been cited that detecting nonverbal cues such as fidgeting, crying, poor hygiene, or signs of intoxication may be more challenging through telehealth and that maintaining eye contact and experiencing disruptions to conversation flow due to technology would be detrimental to care.[23]

Systematic reviews have consistently reported overall high patient satisfaction with interventions delivered via telehealth.[4,24,25] High patient satisfaction with individual telehealth for behavioral health care has continued to be reported now that it has become the nearly exclusive method of delivering behavioral health care since the COVID-19 pandemic.[26,27] Comparable therapeutic alliance has also been reported when comparing in-person vs. telemental health care.[28] Further, systematic reviews have found additional support that therapeutic alliances are equally strong when care is delivered via telehealth as compared with in-person psychotherapy.[25,29] An interesting new factor to consider in the delivery of in-person behavioral health care is the impact that mask-wearing may have on the therapeutic alliance. Future research will help determine any potential differences in the therapeutic alliance between mask-wearing during in-person visits compared with telehealth for behavioral health.

Behavioral Health Conditions Addressed in Primary Care

PCPs are in a unique position to provide better mental health care and in fact, are one of the main sources of mental health care.[3] Up to 70% of primary care visits are related to a mental health condition.[30] PCPs manage many acute and chronic behavioral health conditions including depressive disorders, anxiety disorders, panic attacks, stress disorders, bipolar disorders, attention deficit hyperactivity disorder, and substance abuse.

Mental health needs have increased during the COVID-19 pandemic, particularly in vulnerable populations.[31,32] Pandemic-related stress has resulted in poorer sleep and eating habits, more difficulties managing chronic conditions, isolation, depression, anxiety, and substance use, and with that increased barriers to care, which could result in an estimated 75,000 additional deaths by suicide and alcohol or drug misuse if we cannot address the behavioral health impact of the pandemic.[33]

According to the CDC, specifically, younger adults, racial/ethnic minorities, essential workers, and unpaid adult caregivers reported having experienced disproportionately worse mental health outcomes, increased substance use, and elevated suicidal ideation:

- 13.3% reported starting or increasing the use of substances[33]
- 40.9% reported at least one adverse mental or behavioral health condition[33]
- 30.9% reported symptoms of anxiety or depression[33]
- 26.3% reported trauma- and stressor-related symptoms related to the pandemic[33]
- 10.7% reported seriously considering suicide 30 days before completing the survey[33]

Of these respondents, symptom rates were significantly higher among respondents:

- Aged 18 to 24 years: 25.5%
- Hispanic respondents: 18.6%
- Non-Hispanic black respondents: 15.1%
- Self-reported unpaid caregivers for adults: 30.7%
- Essential workers: 21.7%[33,34]

Since the pandemic began, an estimated 1.5 million children lost a caregiver, and many more have suffered similar traumatic experiences. There have been a greater number of caregivers lost to COVID-19 in Black, Indigenous, People of Color (BIPOC) communities, and it was recently published that "Black children are disproportionately affected, comprising only 14% of children in the United States but 20% of those losing a parent to COVID-19."[35]

The need for behavioral health services is growing, and when primary care integrates behavioral health services for in-person, virtual, and telephonic care, there is a pathway for increased access promptly; this expands the behavioral health services PCPs can provide their patients.

Behavioral Health Home Monitoring Tools

At the start of the pandemic, the world focused on physical health. Due to safety concerns, practitioners encouraged patients to track physical health using at-home monitoring tools (eg, pulse oximeters, at-home COVID-19 tests, and so forth). It has become apparent that mental health home-monitoring tools are comparably important. At-home behavioral health monitoring measures facilitate the observation of progress in terms of treatment goals. These tools can also inform the patient about their progress as well as any impact on treatment expectations. For example, by completing a bi-weekly patient health questionnaire[36] patients and practitioners can determine progress around alleviating depressive symptomology. Below are some ways to monitor mental health from home:

- Evidence-based measures sent and completed via the electronic health record
  For example, practitioners may send PHQ-9 forms to patients through an EHR
  to be completed before the session, which may allow the practitioner to understand the patient's current symptoms, thus informing the focus of the telehealth
  meeting.
- Patient-driven device applications (Goldberg and colleagues, 2022)
  ○ There are a variety of free and paid apps that can help patients monitor:
    - Mood
    - Drug and alcohol use
    - Meditation sessions
    - Food intake/nutrition
    - Sleep
    - Thoughts
- Wearable fitness trackers
  ○ Fitness tracker information can support the facilitation of treatment goals

While results are generally mixed on the effectiveness of apps in promoting health behavior, reducing health-risk behavior, and improving mood, apps are still a viable home monitoring tool for patients if electronic tracking is their preferred method, as opposed to worksheet tracking.[37] Milne-Ives et. al, 2020 analyzed 52 randomized, controlled trials measuring patient perception and behavioral change based on the use of applications. They found that, while patient perceptions were generally positive, these applications overall did not contribute to significant behavioral changes or improved health outcomes. Despite this, applications can be helpful tools for patient engagement and tracking progress via telehealth.

Benefits of Virtual Behavioral Health

There are multiple benefits to using telehealth for behavioral health concerns in the primary care setting at the system level, the provider level, as well as at the individual patient level.

Benefits of telehealth for behavioral health at the system level

At the system level, there is a potential for overall cost-effectiveness in both increasing capacity to provide more care to patients and reducing expenditures necessary for in-person care (eg, transportation, work hours lost).[4] Telemental health services have also been associated with long-term cost savings including reduced psychiatric hospitalizations, reduced days spent in the hospital, and improved treatment compliance and outcomes.[38]

Offering telehealth to patients maintains a healthy workforce to be able to continue providing care during a much-needed time. Maintaining social distancing during the COVID-19 pandemic and reducing the risk of transmission allows for a safe environment in which behavioral health clinicians can practice.[39] Behavioral health visits typically last longer than primary care visits, and due to the nature of these visits, it is not uncommon for patients to become tearful, take off their mask to blow their nose, have an ill-fitting mask, or have symptoms of COVID-19 that would prevent them from being seen in the clinic.

The flexibility of telehealth delivery can also support the expansion of the behavioral health workforce within primary care, where space is not a concern and providers can flex their schedules to provide overlapping in-person and remote availability. Due to the ability to engage in virtual behavioral health visits wherever a patient may be, decreased no-shows and cancelations also provide additional access to patient care and revenue for practices.[40]

Benefits of telehealth for behavioral health at the provider level

An initial review of the literature examining provider benefits of a transition to telehealth for behavioral health services indicates several factors that providers appreciate. This includes greater work-life balance for individuals who prefer the opportunity to work remotely or need to for childcare reasons. These providers now have the flexibility of continuing to see patients virtually rather than having to cancel and reschedule,[41] have increased schedule flexibility,[42] lack a commute,[43] and have reduced burnout.[44]

Telehealth with patients in their homes also offers additional contextual data that can enhance care. This may include having access to the home environment to get a better sense of patients' struggles, be it their sleep environment to address sleep hygiene concerns, whereby medications are stored and how they are organized to promote treatment adherence, opportunities to engage within vivo exposure in the home environment whereby patients are coming in to contact with potentially anxiety-provoking stimuli, engaging in safety planning with family support who may also be available in the home, or observing pets or toys as a means to connect and build rapport.[45]

Benefits of telehealth for behavioral health at the patient level

Multiple benefits of telehealth are reported at the patient level. Increased access, affordability by way of reducing expenditures to attend an in-person appointment, (eg, not needing to take time away from work to drive to and from an appointment, not needing to facilitate childcare coverage), and transportation barriers are commonly mentioned in the literature.[46] During the COVID-19 pandemic, patients with comorbid physical health and mental health concerns may prefer to be seen virtually to avoid possible exposure to illness. Telehealth also has the advantages to reach individuals in rural areas who may otherwise have limited access to providers[47] as well as providing support to those feeling isolated in their homes. Telehealth may also help to reduce stigma for individuals who have been hesitant to come to in-person behavioral health services.[48] Patient satisfaction with telehealth for behavioral health services has been consistently reported as high across multiple populations including perinatal patients, older adults, children, and general adult populations.[27,49–51]

Barriers to Virtual Behavioral Health Care

There are also many barriers to using telehealth for behavioral health concerns in the primary care setting at the system level, the provider level, as well as at the individual patient level.

Barriers to telehealth for behavioral health at the system level

The utilization of telehealth services had been incorporated slowly into medical systems before the pandemic despite literature suggesting the potential benefit of administering care in this manner.[46] From a systems level, some of the slow integration of telehealth services have been attributed to reimbursement concerns, policy regulations, and the cost of telehealth infrastructure.

Parity is needed to ensure that providers will receive comparable reimbursement for telehealth encounters as they would in-person visits as well as ensure that coverage would be guaranteed for telehealth services. Before the COVID-19 pandemic, only a handful of states had telehealth parity laws making telehealth services a much less desirable and feasible investment to make.[52] To further complicate the picture, no 2 states have the same definition or regulation of telehealth services, which can narrow accessibility to these visits depending on who the service provider is, which insurance coverage is used, the type of electronic service provided, and the patient's location when receiving the service.[53] Inconsistent and inadequate reimbursement for telehealth services continues to plague efforts by institutions, organizations, and systems to implement the delivery of telemedicine to patients.[46] Regarding policy regulations, the COVID-19 pandemic prompted policymakers and insurers to make telehealth services rapidly available; however, it remains to be seen what future policy, concerning telehealth services, will look like.[54,55] The financial costs of implementing telehealth infrastructure also play a role in the uptake of services. Waugh, Voyles, and Thomas[46] referenced several cost types including fixed (videoconferencing technology), variable (connectivity, hardware, clinic space, personnel), opportunity (possibility for disagreement between a provider's service hours and billable hours), and reimbursable (dependent on payer source and service type), highlighting the complexity of implementing telehealth on a large scale.

It is clear that there are several system-level barriers to implementing telehealth services, and while systems are attempting to improve the availability and equity of health care services via telehealth platforms, researchers have also stressed the importance of ensuring telehealth services are provided in an equitable and accessible manner given that there is a real risk of further contributing to the "digital divide in which populations that have poorer health outcomes continue to have poorer health outcomes despite technological improvements" (p. 1).[56] Ensuring that the implementation of telehealth services does not exacerbate or perpetuate poor health outcomes and inequities in health care need to be considered carefully when designing and executing a largely new method of patient care.[54,56,57]

Barriers to telehealth for behavioral health at the provider level

Before the COVID-19 pandemic, the proportion of behavioral health services administered via telehealth was small.[58] However, the adoption of telehealth services by psychologists increased rapidly at the beginning of the COVID-19 crisis.[59] Given that providing telehealth services was uncommon prepandemic, formal training on telehealth practices had not been included in accreditation standards for mental health providers meaning that individual clinicians might not be adequately prepared to deliver culturally sensitive and in-person equivalent standards of care.[58]

An overall lack of formal training for providers administering telehealth services can be a limiting factor in providing this type of treatment. Prior research suggests clinicians' technological skillset is an important element in providing this type of care from a patient's perspective.[60] When behavioral health services rapidly shifted to being conducted mainly electronically, the boundaries and norms of care also changed. One important example of the changing therapeutic landscape involved informed consent. Informed consent ensures the patient participates in treatment with the knowledge and awareness of the risks/benefits, nature, and course of care (American Psychological Association Standard 3.01, Standard 10.01).[61] In the realm of telehealth, special attention to the changes in the informed consent process need to be considered including clinicians being able to verify a patient's identity, the potential privacy concerns of conducting treatment on virtual platforms and in less confidential locations as well as the potential interruptions with technical glitches or failures.

Barriers to telehealth for behavioral health at the patient level

To respond to the COVID-19 pandemic, behavioral health providers promptly began providing telehealth services to both new and existing patients. In Colorado, legislation was enacted that did not permit carriers offering telehealth services to impose additional training or certifications on providers delivering this method of service as a condition of reimbursement, require there to be an established relationship among a patient and provider, or require the use of specific HIPAA-compliant technologies to deliver these services (see Senate Bill 20–212). This meant that patients were quickly able to access behavioral health services at a time when patients were unable or unwilling to obtain care through in-person settings. While expanding the availability of telehealth provided increased access and continuity of care, it also has the potential to negatively impact health equity for patients.[54,56,57] For instance, since 2019, home broadband subscriptions and Smartphone possession have both increased. However, even with the increased growth of technology, 30% of adults report Internet connectivity issues either often or sometimes, and for individuals without access to broadband home Internet, financial constraints are cited as a primary reason they do not have this service.[62]

Comfort with using telehealth platforms should be individually assessed since each patient will likely differ in his or her ability or proficiency with telehealth platforms. For instance, adaptive devices for patients with disabilities and interpretation services for nonnative speakers could provide significant barriers to receiving telehealth care. In addition to connectivity and access concerns, there are concerns regarding patient privacy.[58,63] For example, behavioral health services have the potential to include a discussion of more personal and sensitive topics that require a private location/space to conduct a visit, which can be challenging for some patients. For patients attending video sessions in the privacy of their homes or personal spaces, it is also important for providers to ensure patients feel comfortable and capable with this method of service provision.[58]

Best Practices for Virtual Behavioral Health Care

Virtual behavioral health care provides an opportunity to integrate behavioral health services immediately into primary care practices. This allows the behavioral health team to be present without requiring them to be physically present in the practice. It also allows the PCP, behavioral health provider, and patient to be in different locations while joined together virtually. Immediate warm hand-offs, connecting a patient to behavioral health practitioners in real-time, can happen anytime regardless of physical location. The behavioral health provider can also receive warm hand-offs from multiple different clinical sites, improving access to care.

The PCP may identify the need for behavioral health care at multiple points in the visit, including:

- The reason for the visit may be a new or uncontrolled mental health issue
- Screening and intake forms including social history documentation, the PHQ screening, or Edinburgh Postnatal Depression Scale, may identify a need for behavioral health care such as new depression or anxiety, a substance use disorder, or acute stressor
- The discussion between the PCP and patient may reveal an acute mental health crisis or need for better control of chronic mental health conditions

A virtual warm hand-off allows the provider to immediately introduce the patient to the behavioral health team. This can be conducted before the office visit if a need is known, during the office visit (eg, through secure text-based communication, joining a visit virtually, or a phone call), or after the office visit once the PCP has finished the appointment.[64]

It is important to recognize that some patients may not be suitable candidates for virtual behavioral health. This may include if the patient:

- Is having an acute psychotic episode
- Is actively suicidal or homicidal

- Does not feel comfortable with virtual communication
- Does not have access to broadband services
- Has a disability limiting virtual health capability
- Has a language barrier, and no translator is available
- Does not have access to a confidential space
- Is a victim of abuse with the potential for the abuser to be present

Alternatively, virtual behavioral health can greatly increase access for individuals who:

- Are responsible for caretaking for young children or elderly[65]
- May be immunocompromised
- Struggle with lack of transportation
- Have busy schedules and cannot afford to take time to travel to the clinic, park, and meet with a psychologist for a full session
- Struggle with agoraphobia or other behavioral health concerns that make travel difficult
- Struggle with a disability or other physical health concerns that make travel difficult

Best practices for integrating virtual behavioral health care into primary care practices include:

- HIPAA-compliant technology
- Process for virtual warm hand-offs (secure chat, phone, and so forth)
- Handling unsafe situations such as suicidal patients
- Building a team of therapists to provide access to the care needed

Once a patient's behavioral health needs have been identified by a PCP, the PCP should reach out to the behavioral health provider. The behavioral health provider and PCP connect using a variety of methods. These include texting, telephone calls, using the "chat" function on medical health record software, or using other HIPAA compliant applications/platforms.

Once the PCP and behavioral health provider connect, they briefly discuss the patient's key behavioral health concerns and create a preliminary course of care. The behavioral health provider then connects directly with the patient and PCP. This connection can take place via various HIPAA-compliant platforms, including through the organization's electronic health record and compatible apps/websites. At this time, a warm handoff is performed, wherein the PCP introduces the patient and behavioral health provider in real-time. There are several options for in vivo behavioral health care once the behavioral health provider and patient connect. Warm handoffs can be nonbillable, focused on an introduction to available services and/or behavioral health triage, or they can be billable, focused on using a specific intervention to address the patient's behavioral health needs in vivo.

For example, if a patient is struggling with primary insomnia, the behavioral health provider may implement psychoeducation, or provide education and support to a patient around psychological factors. Psychoeducation around how to enact sleep hygiene techniques and assisting the patient in identifying behavioral changes she can make to develop sleep hygiene skills would be appropriate warm hand-off interventions. Alternatively, in a nonbillable warm handoff, the behavioral health provider may triage the patient, assisting her with connecting to a community-based long-term therapist who specializes in the patient's main behavioral health concerns. Warm handoffs can also be facilitated by other medical staff, including medical assistants and nurses if

Table 1		
APA's telepsychology guidelines, rationale, and examples of how they may be applied		
Guideline	**Rationale**	**Specific Example(s) of Application**
(1) Competence of the Psychologist	As telepsychology is an emerging area, psychologists must continuously assess their own competency and risk management practices.	Psychologists should assess and develop their technical competence *in addition to* their regular professional practice competence. Be familiar with local emergency services and prepare a written plan and instructions for patients in case of risk.
(2) Standards of Care in the Delivery of Telepsychology Services	The same ethical and professional standards of care for in-person services must be upheld for telepsychology services. Assessment of the appropriateness of telepsychology technologies is encouraged.	Conduct a risk-benefit analysis of telepsychology services with the consideration of patient's unique characteristics and communicate those with the patient. Consider the efficacy, privacy, and safety of the chosen telepsychology intervention and technology/platform.
(3) Informed Consent	Obtain informed consent by including a thorough description of telepsychology services, policies, and procedures. Also consider implementing additional security measures and inform patients about them.	Obtain and document written informed consent that is specific to the type of services provided. Include boundaries and procedures in the use of technologies. Include billing documentation and fees as part of informed consent as it pertains to specific telepsychology services (eg, video chat, texting fees, and so forth).
(4) Confidentiality	Psychologists must familiarize themselves with risks to confidentiality unique to telepsychology and consult technology experts when needed. Further, psychologists must be thoughtful about boundary issues that may arise from participation in social networking sites.	Consider the risks and benefits of searching patients on the Internet before and during services. Set and maintain appropriate boundaries. Understand the risks to privacy and confidentiality when using electronic communication.
(5) Security and Transmission of Data and Information	Psychologists must be mindful of security threats (eg, hackers, theft, viruses, and so forth) and take steps to protect themselves and patients against them.	Conduct an analysis of security risk - and consult experts when necessary—to ensure data are accessible only by authorized entities and/or individuals.

(continued on next page)

Table 1 (continued)		
Guideline	**Rationale**	**Specific Example(s) of Application**
		When documenting, specify the types of telecommunications used.
(6) Disposal of Data and Information and Technologies	Psychologists must ensure the secure destruction of patient information, particularly electronic data and information and the technologies involved in maintaining that data.	Understand means of storage and disposal of patient data specific to telepsychology technologies (eg, videoconferencing file storage). Document the procedures followed for both storage, transmission, and disposal of data.
(7) Testing and Assessment	Psychologists must consider the suitability of assessments created for in-person use when applying them in telepsychology services. Further, they should maintain the integrity of the original assessment as much as possible.	Maintain the integrity of the original assessment as much as possible. Make and document modifications to testing when needed. Consider all types of possible distractions during assessment (eg, smell, sound, and so forth), and interpret assessment results accordingly. Be aware of special considerations when working with diverse populations (eg, age, physical/sensory impairment, and so forth), and enlist an on-site proctor to facilitate the assessment if needed.
(8) Interjurisdictional Practice	Psychologists must inform themselves of laws and regulations that govern the provision of telepsychology as described by their organizational system, state, province, territory, and country.	When practicing in jurisdictions without laws and regulations in place, search for statements and regulations in relevant governing bodies and nearby jurisdictions to guide telepsychology service delivery. Stay informed of the changes in laws, regulations, and the credentialing of telepsychology as this mode of delivery evolves.

Data from American Psychological Association (APA). 2013. Guidelines for the Practice of Telepsychology. Accessed December 14, 2021. https://www.apa.org/practice/guidelines/telepsychology.

the PCP must move on to the next patient. The behavioral health provider then closes the loop by reporting the outcome of the warm handoff to the PCP. Again, this can be achieved via several online/virtual platforms. Well-staffed clinics may be able to provide patient warm handoffs with behavioral health providers as well as psychiatrists, care managers, social workers, and trainees at all levels.[66]

In response to the fast-changing landscape of behavioral health service delivery via telehealth platforms, scientific and professional organizations representing psychology, psychiatry, and telemedicine could be used as valuable guides for best practices in telehealth.[67,68] The guidelines of the American Psychological Association are informed by psychological theory, evidence-based practice, and multicultural guidelines and considerations. The guidelines apply to the use of all technologies to deliver behavioral health services. Both the psychologists' knowledge and telepsychology competency, as well as the patients' understanding of the increased security and confidentiality risks, should be prioritized. Additionally, the guidelines highlight the importance of inter-jurisdictional practice and encourage psychologists to learn and comply with laws and regulations on inter-jurisdictional and international practice. **Table 1** lists each of the guidelines, their rationale, and examples of how they may be applied.

The American Psychiatric Association and American Telemedicine Association similarly outline their best practices[68] and include many of the same guidelines as the American Psychological Association. Additional considerations by these governing institutions are provided as well. Suggestions are outlined to behavioral health care providers related to program development and administration, communication with patients, and guidelines specific to patient populations and types of providers.

Additional guidelines related to program development and administration include encouragement to providers to obtain malpractice insurance that covers telehealth practices if that coverage is not already included in the current insurance package. Providers should conduct a program development analysis before delivering telehealth services, during which needs related to training, space, types of services, and other administrative considerations are assessed. Additionally, the APA asserts that organizations providing telemental health services should create Standard Operating Procedures that include components such as a quality improvement plan and a method for documenting provider credentials.[68]

The APA offers several directives regarding patient and provider communication, as well. For example, they suggest developing a standard way of identifying both the patient and the telemental health providers(s) present. To do so, the provider might state their name, credentials, and contact information and request that the patient provides their name, location, and contact information at the start of the session.[68] Further, it would be prudent to discuss continued means of communication and emergency management between appointments.[68] The provider should encourage each patient to choose a consistent location whereby they can receive telehealth services to manage risk and maintain an appropriate plan for emergencies.[68] Behavioral health care providers might also assess the patient to determine if an in-person physical examination is needed. If so, the provider must assist the patient in arranging an onsite appointment.[68] Finally, providers are instructed to maintain open communication regarding the wellbeing of the patient with other health care providers as indicated and allowed by local and federal law and privacy guidelines.[68]

SUMMARY

The COVID-19 pandemic has highlighted the growing need for more behavioral health care services, particularly those integrated into the primary care setting whereby many patients first present with mental health needs. We continue to learn more about the barriers and challenges to virtual behavioral health care, while also seeing more data supporting virtual behavioral health care to successfully increase access to mental health services in a timely and effective manner.

CLINICS CARE POINTS

- When considering if a behavioral health visit should occur via telehealth versus in-person, with a few notable exceptions, this can be driven largely by patient preference, as telehealth is as effective as in-person care in delivering high-quality behavioral health services.

- When providing behavioral health care via telehealth, providers should consult the American Psychological Association and American Psychiatric Association standards of care to ensure they are providing ethical, quality care via this rapidly evolving mode of delivery.

ACKNOWLEDGMENTS

The authors would like to thank Elizabeth W. Staton, MSTC from the University of Colorado Department of Family Medicine who helped with editing and formatting the article.

DISCLOSURE

The authors have nothing to disclose.

REFERENCES

1. Panchal N, Kamal R, Cox C, et al. The implications of COVID-19 for mental health and substance use. 2021. Available at: https://www.kff.org/coronavirus-covid-19/issue-brief/the-implications-of-covid-19-for-mental-health-and-substance-use/. accessed December 14 2021).
2. National Institute of Mental Health. Mental illness. Available at: https://www.nimh.nih.gov/health/statistics/mental-illness. accessed December 14 2021.
3. Xierali IM, Tong ST, Petterson SM, et al. Family physicians are essential for mental health care delivery. J Am Board Fam Med 2013;26:114–5.
4. Hilty DM, Ferrer DC, Parish MB, et al. The effectiveness of telemental health: a 2013 review. Telemed J E Health 2013;19:444–54.
5. Knierim K, Palmer C, Kramer ES, et al. Lessons learned during COVID-19 that can move telehealth in primary care forward. J Am Board Fam Med 2021;34:S196–202.
6. Moreno C, Wykes T, Galderisi S, et al. How mental health care should change as a consequence of the COVID-19 pandemic. Lancet Psychiatry 2020;7:813–24.
7. Backhaus A, Agha Z, Maglione ML, et al. Videoconferencing psychotherapy: a systematic review. Psychol Serv 2012;9:111–31.
8. Langarizadeh M, Tabatabaei MS, Tavakol K, et al. Telemental health care, an effective alternative to conventional mental care: a systematic review. Acta Inform Med 2017;25:240–6.
9. Pierce BS, Perrin PB, Tyler CM, et al. The COVID-19 telepsychology revolution: a national study of pandemic-based changes in U.S. mental health care delivery. Am Psychol 2021;76:14–25.

10. Pierce BS, Perrin PB, McDonald SD. Pre-COVID-19 deterrents to practicing with videoconferencing telepsychology among psychologists who didn't. Psychol Serv 2020. https://doi.org/10.1037/ser0000435.

11. Young KS. An empirical examination of client attitudes towards online counseling. Cyberpsychol Behav 2005;8:172–7.

12. Zhai Y. A call for addressing barriers to telemedicine: health disparities during the COVID-19 pandemic. Psychother Psychosom 2021;90:64–6.

13. Ramsetty A, Adams C. Impact of the digital divide in the age of COVID-19. J Am Med Inform Assoc 2020;27:1147–8.

14. United States Veterans Affairs. VA expands telehealth by allowing health care providers to treat patients across state lines. 2018. Available at: https://www.va.gov/opa/pressrel/pressrelease.cfm?id=4054. accessed 11/29 2021.

15. Centers for Medicare & Medicaid Services. Medicare telemedicine health care provider fact sheet. 2020. Available at: https://www.cms.gov/newsroom/fact-sheets/medicare-telemedicine-health-care-provider-fact-sheet.   accessed September 25 2020).

16. National Association of Behavioral Healthcare. CMS expands medicare telehealth coverage for mental health and addiction treatment services. 2021. Available at: https://www.nabh.org/cms-expands-medicare-telehealth-coverage-for-mental-health-and-addiction-treatment-services. accessed 11/29 2021).

17. Health Resources & Services Administration. Best practice guide: telehealth for behavioral health care. 2021. Available at: https://telehealth.hhs.gov/providers/telehealth-for-behavioral-health/billing-for-telebehavioral-health. accessed 11/29 2021.

18. Berryhill MB, Culmer N, Williams N, et al. Videoconferencing psychotherapy and depression: a systematic review. Telemed J E Health 2019;25:435–46.

19. Fernandez E, Woldgabreal Y, Day A, et al. Live psychotherapy by video versus in-person: a meta-analysis of efficacy and its relationship to types and targets of treatment. Clin Psychol Psychother 2021. https://doi.org/10.1002/cpp.2594.

20. Frueh BC, Monnier J, Yim E, et al. A randomized trial of telepsychiatry for post-traumatic stress disorder. J Telemed Telecare 2007;13:142–7.

21. Mitchell JE, Crosby RD, Wonderlich SA, et al. Randomized trial comparing the efficacy of cognitive-behavioral therapy for bulimia nervosa delivered via telemedicine versus face-to-face. Behav Res Ther 2008;46:581–92.

22. Morland LA, Greene CJ, Rosen CS, et al. Telemedicine for anger management therapy in a rural population of combat veterans with posttraumatic stress disorder: a randomized noninferiority trial. J Clin Psychiatry 2010;71:855–63.

23. Connolly SL, Miller CJ, Lindsay JA, et al. A systematic review of providers' attitudes toward telemental health via videoconferencing. Clin Psychol-sci Pr 2020;27. https://doi.org/10.1111/cpsp.12311.

24. Richardson LK, Frueh BC, Grubaugh AL, et al. Current directions in videoconferencing tele-mental health research. Clin Psychol (New York) 2009;16:323–38.

25. Jenkins-Guarnieri MA, Pruitt LD, Luxton DD, et al. Patient perceptions of telemental health: systematic review of direct comparisons to in-person psychotherapeutic treatments. Telemed E-Health 2015;21:652–60.

26. Sugarman DE, Busch AB, McHugh RK, et al. Patients' perceptions of telehealth services for outpatient treatment of substance use disorders during the COVID-19 pandemic. Am J Addict 2021;30:445–52.

27. Guinart D, Marcy P, Hauser M, et al. Patient attitudes toward telepsychiatry during the COVID-19 pandemic: a nationwide, multisite survey. JMIR Ment Health 2020;7:e24761.

28. Stiles-Shields C, Kwasny MJ, Cai X, et al. Therapeutic alliance in face-to-face and telephone-administered cognitive behavioral therapy. J Consult Clin Psychol 2014;82:349–54.

29. Sucala M, Schnur JB, Constantino MJ, et al. The therapeutic relationship in e-therapy for mental health: a systematic review. J Med Internet Res 2012;14:e110.

30. Hunter CL, Goodie JL, Oordt MS, et al. Integrated behavioral health in primary care: step-by-step guidance for assessment and intervention. Washington, DC, US: American Psychological Association; 2009. p. 291.

31. Han B, Compton WM, Blanco C, et al. Prevalence, treatment, and unmet treatment needs of us adults with mental health and substance use disorders. Health Aff (Millwood) 2017;36:1739–47.

32. Diaz A, Baweja R, Bonatakis JK, et al. Global health disparities in vulnerable populations of psychiatric patients during the COVID-19 pandemic. World J Psychiatry 2021;11:94–108.

33. Czeisler ME, Lane RI, Petrosky E, et al. Mental health, substance use, and suicidal ideation during the COVID-19 pandemic - United States, June 24-30, 2020. MMWR-Morb Mortal Wkly Rep 2020;69:1049–57.

34. Substance Abuse and Mental Health Services Administration. Key substance use and mental health indicators in the United States: results from the 2019 national survey on drug use and health. 2020. HHS Publication No. PEP20-07-01-001, NSDUH Series H-55). Available at: https://www.samhsa.gov/data/sites/default/files/reports/rpt29393/2019NSDUHFFRPDFWHTML/2019NSDUHFFR090120.htm. accessed December 14 2021.

35. Kidman R, Margolis R, Smith-Greenaway E, et al. Estimates and Projections of COVID-19 and Parental Death in the US. JAMA Pediatr 2021;175:745–6.

36. Kroenke K, Spitzer RL, Williams JB. The PHQ-9: validity of a brief depression severity measure. J Gen Intern Med 2001;16:606–13.

37. Milne-Ives M, Lam C, De Cock C, et al. Mobile apps for health behavior change in physical activity, diet, drug and alcohol use, and mental health: systematic review. JMIR Mhealth and Uhealth 2020;8. https://doi.org/10.2196/17046.

38. Godleski L, Darkins A, Peters J. Outcomes of 98,609 U.S. department of veterans affairs patients enrolled in telemental health services, 2006-2010. Psychiatr Serv 2012;63:383–5.

39. Madigan S, Racine N, Cooke JE, et al. COVID-19 and telemental health: benefits, challenges, and future directions. Can Psychol 2021;62:5–11.

40. Mishkind MC, Shore JH, Bishop K, et al. Rapid conversion to telemental health services in response to COVID-19: experiences of two outpatient mental health clinics. Telemed E-Health 2021;27:778–84.

41. Yellowlees P, Nakagawa K, Pakyurek M, et al. Rapid conversion of an outpatient psychiatric clinic to a 100% virtual telepsychiatry clinic in response to COVID-19. Psychiatr Serv 2020;71:749–52.

42. Siegel A, Zuo Y, Moghaddamcharkari N, et al. Barriers, benefits and interventions for improving the delivery of telemental health services during the coronavirus disease 2019 pandemic: a systematic review. Curr Opin Psychiatry 2021;34:434–43.

43. Steidtmann D, McBride S, Mishkind MC. Experiences of mental health clinicians and staff in rapidly converting to full-time telemental health and work from home during the COVID-19 pandemic. Telemed E-Health 2021;27:785–91.

44. Gardner JS, Plaven BE, Yellowlees P, et al. Remote telepsychiatry workforce: a solution to psychiatry's workforce issues. Curr Psychiatry Rep 2020;22:8.

45. Pruitt LD, Luxton DD, Shore P. Additional clinical benefits of home-based tele-mental health treatments. Psychol Serv 2014;45:340–6.
46. Waugh M, Voyles D, Thomas MR. Telepsychiatry: benefits and costs in a changing health-care environment. Int Rev Psychiatry 2015;27:558–68.
47. Benavides-Vaello S, Strode A, Sheeran BC. Using technology in the delivery of mental health and substance abuse treatment in rural communities: a review. J Behav Health Serv Res 2013;40:111–20.
48. Olden M, Cukor J, Rizzo AS, et al. House calls revisited: leveraging technology to overcome obstacles to veteran psychiatric care and improve treatment outcomes. Ann N Y Acad Sci 2010;1208:133–41.
49. Ackerman M, Greenwald E, Noulas P, et al. Patient satisfaction with and use of telemental health services in the perinatal period: a survey study. Psychiatr Q 2021;92:925–33.
50. Hantke N, Lajoy M, Gould CE, et al. Patient satisfaction with geriatric psychiatry services via video teleconference. Am J Geriatr Psychiatry 2020;28:491–4.
51. Mayworm AM, Lever N, Gloff N, et al. School-based telepsychiatry in an urban setting: efficiency and satisfaction with care. Telemed E-Health 2020;26:446–54.
52. Warren JC, Smalley BK. Using telehealth to meet mental health needs during the covid-19 crisis. To the Point (blog). 2020. Available at: https://doi.org/10.26099/qb81-6c84. accessed December 14 2021.
53. Center for Connected Health Policy. State telehealth laws and Medicaid program policies. 2021. Available at: https://www.cchpca.org/2021/10/Fall2021_ExecutiveSummary_FINAL.pdf. accessed December 14 2021.
54. Cantor JH, McBain RK, Pera MF, et al. Who is (and is not) receiving telemedicine care during the COVID-19 pandemic. Am J Prev Med 2021;61:434–8.
55. Lucia K, Blumberg LJ, Curran E. The COVID-19 pandemic – insurer insights into challenges, implications, and lessons learned. 2020. Available at: https://www.urban.org/research/publication/covid-19-pandemic-insurer-insights-challenges-implications-and-lessons-learned. accessed November 30 2021).
56. Saeed SA, Masters RM. Disparities in health care and the digital divide. Curr Psychiatry Rep 2021;23:61.
57. Chunara R, Zhao Y, Chen J, et al. Telemedicine and healthcare disparities: a cohort study in a large healthcare system in New York City during COVID-19. J Am Med Inform Assoc 2020;28:33–41.
58. Comer JS. Rebooting mental health care delivery for the COVID-19 pandemic (and beyond): guiding cautions as telehealth enters the clinical mainstream. Cogn Behav Pract 2021;28:743–8.
59. Sammons MT, VandenBos GR, Martin JN, et al. Psychological practice at six months of COVID-19: a follow-up to the first national survey of psychologists during the pandemic. J Health Serv Psychol 2020;1–10.
60. Henry BW, Block DE, Ciesla JR, et al. Clinician behaviors in telehealth care delivery: a systematic review. Adv Health Sci Education 2017;22:869–88.
61. American Psychological Association. Ethical principles of psychologists and code of conduct. 2017. https://www.apa.org/ethics/code/ethics-code-2017.pdf. accessed December 14 2021.
62. Perrin A. Mobile Technology and Home Broadband 2021. 2021. Available at: https://www.pewresearch.org/internet/2021/06/03/mobile-technology-and-home-broadband-2021/. accessed December 14 2021.
63. Crockett JL, Becraft JL, Phillips ST, et al. Rapid conversion from clinic to telehealth behavioral services during the COVID-19 pandemic. Behav Anal Pract 2020;13:725–35.

64. Kanzler KE, Ogbeide S. Addressing trauma and stress in the COVID-19 pandemic: challenges and the promise of integrated primary care. Psychol Trauma 2020;12:S177–9.
65. Fiks AG, Jenssen BP, Ray KN. A defining moment for pediatric primary care tele-health. JAMA Pediatr 2021;175:9–10.
66. Raney L, Bergman D, Torous J, et al. Digitally driven integrated primary care and behavioral health: how technology can expand access to effective treatment. Curr Psychiatry Rep 2017;19. https://doi.org/10.1007/s11920-017-0838-y.
67. American Psychological Association. Guidelines for the practice of telepsychology. 2013. Available at: https://www.apa.org/practice/guidelines/telepsychology. accessed December 14 2021.
68. American Psychiatric Association. Best practices in videoconferencing-based telemental health. 2018. Available at: https://www.psychiatry.org/psychiatrists/practice/telepsychiatry/toolkit/practice-guidelines. accessed December 14 2021.

Telehealth in Geriatrics

Tracy Johns, PharmD*, Charisse Huot, MD, Julia C. Jenkins, MD

KEYWORDS

- Telehealth • Telemedicine • Virtual • Remote • Mobile • Technology • Synchronous
- Older • Geriatrics

KEY POINTS

- Telehealth has demonstrated feasibility for geriatric patient care. Telehealth interventions should be designed with the unique needs of geriatric patients in mind for effective implementation.
- Telemedicine has the potential for synchronous communication between patients, caregivers, primary care providers, and specialists to enhance care coordination.
- Current evidence supports the use of telehealth for remote geriatric assessments including medication review, fall and safety risk, frailty and functional status, and nutritional status.
- Telehealth has applications for chronic disease management in older adults, including dementia, depression, hypertension, diabetes mellitus, and heart failure.
- More research is needed to evaluate health outcomes and cost-effectiveness of telehealth interventions in the geriatric population, which will help guide appropriate reimbursement policies.

INTRODUCTION

Telehealth is now an integral part of health care, although questions remain about its effective utilization in geriatrics. Rising health care costs and increasing numbers of age-related diseases are seen with the continued expansion of our aging population.[1] Lack of transportation may lead to older patients' inability to visit a health care provider's office, particularly in rural areas. Geriatric patients are more likely to have mobility and sensory impairments, increasing their chance of injury when leaving the home.[2,3] Timely, high-quality geriatric care which effectively addresses the above issues is needed, ideally guided by patient-centered medical homes. Virtual home-based visits can improve access to care while also promoting patient safety.[2]

This review presents current evidence for the use of various telehealth applications in the geriatric population. Virtual geriatric clinics have been increasingly used during

University of South Florida Morsani College of Medicine, University of South Florida/Morton Plant Mease Family Medicine Residency, Dr. Joseph A. Eaddy Family Medicine Research Center, Turley Family Health Center, 807 North Myrtle Avenue, Clearwater, FL 33755, USA
* Corresponding author.
E-mail address: Tracy.johns@baycare.org

Prim Care Clin Office Pract 49 (2022) 659–676
https://doi.org/10.1016/j.pop.2022.04.009
0095-4543/22/© 2022 Elsevier Inc. All rights reserved.

the SARS-CoV-2 pandemic.[2] Despite initial widespread use out of necessity, telehealth is now commonly used for comprehensive geriatric assessment, health promotion, and disease management.[2,4] Nonetheless, more data are needed regarding the overall utility of telehealth and impact on health care quality and costs. Health care providers should be aware of new and changing policies for the reimbursement of telehealth services.

In this article, the term telehealth broadly refers to all health care modalities provided at a distance, which may or may not include interaction with a medical provider. Telemedicine refers to video, audio, or written remote clinical encounters between a provider and a patient. Remote patient monitoring (RPM) is the technology that enables providers to monitor patient health data outside of conventional clinic settings. Mobile health (mHealth) is a term for mobile phone applications or other wireless devices that help provide either provider-driven or consumer-driven medical advice. Generally, electronic health (eHealth) is the term used when providers use wireless devices to provide care.[5]

DISCUSSION
Patient Safety

Coordination of care
Virtual geriatric clinics enable geriatricians to collaborate with allied health professions including nursing, pharmacy, home health, and occupational and physical therapy with a high degree of patient and physician satisfaction.[2,4] They enhance the coordination of care across multiple settings, inclusive of the community, nursing home (NH), and hospital, resulting in successful pharmacy reviews and reduced hospitalizations. Interactions with caregivers of older adults can be enhanced with telemedicine, improving communication and quality of care. Telemedicine has the potential for three-way, synchronous communication between patients, caregivers, primary care, and specialists to reconcile potentially conflicting recommendations from different providers.

Assisted-living facility (ALF) and NH virtual care has helped protect vulnerable seniors during the COVID-19 pandemic, and its widespread adoption also highlighted other benefits beyond supporting isolation and contact precautions. In an international meta-analysis of 16 studies from 2014 to 2020, a wide spectrum of ALF and NH telehealth services were shown to have cost savings benefits by using virtual geriatrician and specialist consultations, psychiatric care, wound care, and RPM.[6] Some studies demonstrated reductions in hospitalizations and unnecessary transfers.

Home safety and falls
For in-home patient safety assessments, telemedicine enables providers to directly observe the patient's home environment and visualize the mechanics of their daily activities. Fall screening questionnaires can be used in the telehealth setting.[4] Some mobility assessment tools like the Timed-Up-And-Go-Test are not practical in a virtual encounter, but the validated 30 Second Chair Stand Test can easily be used (**Table 1**). For patients with mobility impairment, assistive devices may be appropriately prescribed. Further evaluation of the interior of the home should be conducted for patients with increased fall risk. A virtual home tour alerts the provider to fall hazards such as stairs, inadequate lighting, loose throw rugs, electrical cords, signs of hoarding, or crowded furniture. Providers should visualize the patient's bedroom and bathroom to determine if there is a need and adequate space for durable medical equipment (DME) like a shower chair, commode seat lift, grab bars, or bedside commode. Home modifications to promote safety and reduce the risk of fall or injury

Table 1			
Summary of telemedicine geriatric assessment (GA) tools			
GA Category	**Traditional GA Tool**	**Telehealth Modified GA Tools and Applications**	**Current Evidence for Use of Telehealth GA**
Home Safety, Mobility, and Falls	Tinetti Performance Oriented Mobility Assessment Timed Up-And-Go Test 30 s Chair Stand Test In-Home Occupational Therapy home safety evaluation	30 s Chair Stand Test Virtual Occupational Therapy home safety evaluation	Virtual home safety assessment conducted by Occupational Therapy is technologically feasible for dementia patients and caregivers[8] Remote home assessments made by home modification experts are feasible and the recommendations made concur with traditional in-home visits[7]
Medication Review	In-person clinician- or pharmacist-led medication review Beers criteria STOPP/START criteria	Telephonic or live synchronous video clinician- or pharmacist-led medication review Beers criteria[50] STOPP/START criteria Direct visualization of pillbox and medicine cabinet	Benefit of pharmacist telephonic medication management in transitional care[11–13] Benefit of polypharmacy management[2] Improved medication rationalization[2] Decreased ER visits, hospitalizations, and readmissions[2,11,12] Reduced clinical alerts and adverse drug events[13]
Functional Status	Katz ADL Scale OARS IADL Scale Fall screening questionnaire	Katz ADL Scale OARS IADL Scale[4] Fall screening questionnaire[4] Electronic or mobile health Interventions	eHealth interventions may increase physical activity (steps/d, min/d of moderate-vigorous activity)[17] Mixed data regarding the use of mHealth apps to increase

(continued on next page)

Table 1
(*continued*)

GA Category	Traditional GA Tool	Telehealth Modified GA Tools and Applications	Current Evidence for Use of Telehealth GA
			physical activity, decrease sedentary time, and improve physical fitness[14–16]
Frailty	Weakness (grip strength, sarcopenia) Gait speed Self-reported low level of physical activity Self-reported exhaustion Unintentional weight loss	Limited - ask patient about perceived weakness or instruct caregiver to perform strength testing Evaluate gait speed if patient/ caregiver able to set up camera Reported low level of physical activity by patient/ caregiver Self-reported exhaustion Ask about perceived weight loss or change in clothing size	Limited data on the feasibility of diagnosing frailty and sarcopenia via telehealth Limitations in telehealth physical examination for frailty/sarcopenia diagnosis[2] Telehealth is useful for the chronic management of frail older adults[3] Remote interventions resulted in improvements in quality of life, mentation, balance, and depression in frail elders[6]
Nutritional Status	Mini Nutritional Assessment BMI, waist circumference	Modified Mini-Nutritional Assessment (omit calf circumference, omit BMI if scale not available)[4,18] BMI (ask about perceived weight loss or change in clothing size if scale not available) 24-h dietary recall Virtual kitchen, dining, and pantry tour Telehealth/ telemonitoring nutritional interventions for older adults	Mixed data regarding telemonitoring nutritional interventions on improved macronutrient intake, quality of life, energy intake, and physical function[18,19]

(*continued on next page*)

		Telehealth Modified GA Tools and	Current Evidence for
Table 1 **(continued)**			
GA Category	**Traditional GA Tool**	**Applications**	**Use of Telehealth GA**
Neuropsychiatric Assessment	MMSE MoCA PHQ-2, PHQ-9 Geriatric Depression Scale	MMSE[24,25] MoCA (original) or MoCA Abbreviated Telephone Version[24,25,36] PHQ-2, PHQ-9[4,24] Geriatric Depression Scale[4,24]	Telehealth is feasible and well accepted for dementia care with mixed data on cognitive outcomes[3,27,28] Reliability of GA tools administered via telehealth is comparable to in-person visits; may be limited by hearing/vision impairment[2,3,24] Videoconferencing and smartphone apps may be useful for dementia patients and caregivers to track clinical progression markers[26] Virtual care is an effective alternative for rural patients with dementia[27,28] Video counseling enhances geriatric depression care in nursing home residents[29] Video psychotherapy is noninferior to in-person psychotherapy for veterans with depression[29]

Abbreviations: ADL, activities of daily living; IADL, instrumental activities of daily living; MMSE, Mini-Mental State Examination; MoCA, montreal cognitive assessment; PHQ-2, Patient Health Questionnaire 2-item; PHQ-9, Patient Health Questionnaire 9-item; STOPP/START, Screening Tool of Older Person's Prescriptions/Screening Tool to Alert to Right Treatment.

can be recommended such as adding or repairing handrails, installing a ramp or lift, or rearranging furniture.[7]

Research shows that real-time home safety evaluations are most effective when delivered by occupational therapists. While telehealth ostensibly offers a view into the patient's living situation, there is little data about the feasibility or challenges of these assessments. A study of 10 Veteran's Administration (VA) dementia patients and their caregivers examined the feasibility of telehealth for occupational therapy home safety assessments.[8] The study evaluated the resource, device, and software requirements of such visits. Technological difficulties occurred in nearly all visits, including total loss of audio using a laptop (50% of visits), periodic loss of audio (70%), audio latency or lag (20%), video pixilation (50%), and freezing of video (40%). Nevertheless, the authors concluded that overall visits were technologically feasible. The study had some limitations affecting the generalizability of the results to practice in other settings. It included a small sample and a racially homogenous population. Additionally, the researchers conducting the study were highly motivated to troubleshoot any problems during visits to ensure their success, with resources and technological support from the VA health system. The study did not evaluate the clinical impact of the telehealth evaluations.

Another study compared 2 types of remote assessments, a "zero-tech" paper-and-pencil protocol and a "high-tech" video conference protocol, to traditional in-home assessments in 73 households.[7] The study aimed to determine if remote assessment was feasible and concurred with in-home assessment by expert home-modification specialists, as evidenced by the effectiveness of each intervention to identify problems and prescribe appropriate solutions. The study showed the rate of correct problem identification was significant for both remote paper-and-pencil (96.4%) and remote video (87.1%) protocols. There was also a high rate of agreement on recommended solutions for both types of remote assessments (78.8% and 77.4%, respectively). This study suggests virtual in-home assessments may have similar efficacy to their traditional in-home counterparts.

Medication review

Medication review via telemedicine provides unique insights that may not be gleaned from an office visit. During a virtual encounter, patients can be asked to show all medications they are taking, which are not always consistent with those reported in the office.[9,10] A study of discrepancies between physician and patient medication lists in older patients showed that 37% of medications were being taken without their family physician's knowledge, 6% were not being taken by patients although their physician thought they were, and 10% had dose or frequency discrepancies, which all increase the likelihood of drug interactions.[9] During a virtual visit, providers should reconcile medications from other clinicians, evaluate how patients to store and organize their medications, visualize pillboxes to assess adherence, and instruct patients to discard old and expired medications.

Benefits of virtual medication management were evaluated in a recent systematic review. Seven studies reported clinical outcomes of geriatric virtual clinics.[2] All the studies were an observational design and heterogeneity was noted with the structure of virtual models. Polypharmacy was one of the outcomes felt to be amenable to assessment with virtual visits. Four studies suggested benefits in medication rationalization. Several studies reported a decrease in emergency department visits and hospitalizations with the reconciliation of polypharmacy.

Resource utilization is a common outcome for studies evaluating telemedicine interventions, particularly in transitional care. Two retrospective studies suggested the benefit of pharmacist telephonic medication reconciliation for older adults discharged from the hospital. Liu and colleagues[11] evaluated a transitional care program in a geriatric clinic. Using claims data, they found significantly higher odds of hospital utilization (OR: 1.69, 95% CI: 1.06–2.68) and inpatient admission (OR: 2.54, 95% CI: 1.18–5.44) within 30 days after discharge for patients receiving usual care versus telephone follow-up. Paquin and colleagues[12] studied a service that included medication reconciliation, safety review, and a telephone call with patients or caregivers. Patients were at high risk of dementia or taking dementia medications. The intervention was associated with a lower likelihood of readmission 60 days after discharge compared with those without a pharmacist call (OR: 0.72, 95% CI: 0.57–0.91) and saved $804 per patient. These 2 studies suggest that telephonic strategies are beneficial and feasible in vulnerable older adults, including those in underserved communities and those at high risk of cognitive impairment.

In a study of NH residents, a pharmacist-led telehealth intervention was compared with usual care.[13] Pharmacists performed medication reconciliation and medication regimen review within 72 hours of admission for patients with high-risk medications, then the evaluation of clinical alerts throughout the resident's stay using video tablet-based telemedicine. Telemedicine was used only if residents were cognitively intact. The intervention resulted in less clinical alerts (2.60 vs 9.52/1000 resident days, $P = .009$) during the residents' stay. There was also a lower incidence of alert-specific adverse drug events (0.14 vs 0.61/1000 resident days, $P = .002$). Telemedicine interaction between residents and pharmacists may have resulted in earlier opportunities to resolve medication-related problems and avoid adverse events.

Remote Health Evaluation

Functional status
Standardized functional status assessment tools such as the Activities of Daily Living and OARS Instrumental Activities of Daily Living scales have been used in telehealth visits (see **Table 1**).[4] Remote assessments alert physicians to mobility and safety issues within the home and enable them to recommend solutions such as DME and home modifications to improve the patient's functional status.[7] Direct observation of the patient's home environment and its impact on their activities of daily living through the telehealth platform may help the provider document medical necessity of equipment or homebound status.

Several types of telehealth interventions have been evaluated regarding physical activity, fitness, and functional capacity in community-dwelling older adults. A systematic review and meta-analysis of studies using mHealth interventions showed in a pooled analysis that mHealth apps may increase physical activity, decrease sedentary time, and improve physical fitness. All but one of the studies were randomized controlled trials (RCTs). There was a high degree of heterogeneity among the studies and effects were not significant.[14] In 5 of the 6 studies, interventions used apps that synced with a separate device. Various attributes of apps in individual studies that seemed to confer more benefit included goal-setting, self-monitoring, instructions for performing the behavior, social reward and support, and risk communication. Two of the more effective interventions used mHealth apps in combination with provider support.[15,16]

Several types of eHealth interventions may increase physical activity in healthy older adults. A systematic review and meta-analysis of 19 studies by Nunes de Arenas-Arroyo and colleagues included RCTs evaluating eHealth interventions.[17] The types of interventions were web-based or through mobile phones. Those that used a website often provided feedback through email or interactive forums. Text messaging and phone calls were used in mobile interventions; one study used a mobile app. Education and goal setting were common elements of interventions. The meta-analysis of 18 studies showed mostly moderate effect sizes and pooled mean increases of approximately 1616 steps/d, 7.4 min/d of moderate-to-vigorous physical activity, 40.5 min/wk of physical activity, 56.4 min/wk of moderate-to-vigorous physical activity. The highest degree of heterogeneity among the studies was related to steps/d and moderate-to-vigorous physical activity measured in min/d. Nonetheless, these results suggest the positive effects of eHealth interventions in promoting physical activity.

Frailty

Objective assessment of weakness and grip strength may be challenging in the telehealth setting. There is concern that the limited physical examination via telemedicine reduces the feasibility of diagnosing important geriatric syndromes.[2] However, some criteria for frailty may be evaluated virtually, such as asking about the patient's perception of fatigue or exhaustion, and decreased level of activity (see **Table 1**). Patients who lack access to a scale may be asked if they have gone down in clothing size to screen for unintentional weight loss. Slow walking speed can be evaluated via video if the patient or caregiver is able to set up the device to capture their gait. Telehealth has been used for the chronic management of frail, community-dwelling older adults. In a scoping review by Doraiswamy and colleagues[3] of 79 studies, 24 articles discussed the use of telehealth for specific disease conditions in geriatric patients. Among these, frailty was the second-most common condition for which telehealth services were used (5/24 studies; 20.8%), following dementia (9/24; 37.5%). Small RCTs of different remote interventions for frail elders have shown improvements in quality of life from video exercises paired with weekly phone calls, mentation from computer-based exercises, balance with home exercise paired with phone calls, and reduced depression from therapy delivered via telehealth.[6] However, there are few studies that directly compare the efficacy of delivery of these services via telehealth with face-to-face delivery.

Nutritional status

Nutritional screening and interventions for under- or overweight and obese seniors have been conducted via live video and remote telemonitoring. Standard tools like the Mini-Nutritional Assessment (MNA) or modified versions can be used (see **Table 1**).[4,18] A virtual pantry assessment by live video connection helps corroborate a forgetful patient's informal dietary recall. It can also give insight into problems like food insecurity that may not be apparent at an office visit, prompting referral to appropriate community resources like Meals on Wheels, food banks, or a social worker. For patients reporting a decline in food intake, touring the layout of the kitchen and dining areas through live synchronous video may help the provider determine if the problem is due to mobility issues or physical impairments that impede food preparation and feeding. Collaboration with caregivers during virtual visits is essential for elders who depend on others for shopping, meal preparation, or feeding.

Data regarding the efficacy of telehealth for nutritional status evaluation and management in older adults are mixed. A telemonitoring nutritional intervention study was conducted on 214 older, community-dwelling Dutch adults.[18] Participants were allocated to control, or intervention groups based on municipality. The 6-month intervention included multi-faceted nutritional telemonitoring, nutrition education, and nurse follow-up. Telemonitoring consisted of patients self-measuring their weight, steps, and blood pressure using a provided scale, pedometer, and sphygmomanometer that displayed results on their television and sent data to nurses via secure connection for review at regular intervals. The authors concluded the intervention improved the nutritional status of patients at risk for poor nutrition and improved dietary intake of some macronutrients and fiber, but did not affect body weight, appetite, physical functioning, or quality of life.

A systematic review and meta-analysis aimed to determine the efficacy of telehealth for delivering nutritional interventions to community-dwelling older adults found different results. Nine studies were included in the analysis; in 2 studies, interventions were delivered to disease-specific groups (kidney disease and cancer), and the remaining 7 included patients with mixed morbidities following inpatient discharge. Telehealth interventions varied and included telephone calls by dieticians and providers at regular intervals; use of a telemonitoring device in which patients entered data about body weight and answered questions about appetite, supplements, well-being, and fluid intake; and use of a tablet-based app to order energy- and protein-enriched meals for delivery to patients following hospital discharge. The interventions resulted in improved protein intake by 0.13 g/kg/d as well as improvements in quality of life, with trends toward improved nutrition status, energy intake, physical function, and clinical outcomes.[19]

Medicare Annual Wellness Visit

Medicare Annual Wellness Visits (AWV) are an important touchpoint to conduct health risk assessments, provide preventive health recommendations, and update screenings for seniors.[20] Data on the full impact of the pandemic on Medicare AWV are still pending, but preliminary studies show a drastic decrease in national breast, cervical, and colorectal cancer screenings.[21] Patterns through April 2020 showed steep declines in cervical and breast cancer screenings by 94%, and in colorectal cancer screening by 86%.[22] Screenings that require in-person visits decreased by 91% between March and June 2020.[22,23] In comparison, screening by home-based tests like the multi-targeted stool-based colorectal screening test (Cologuard) and fecal immunochemical test (FIT) decreased to a lesser degree (65% and 87%, respectively).

The Medicare AWV (both initial and subsequent) are permitted via telemedicine by the Centers for Medicare and Medicaid Services (CMS) and their adoption could ameliorate the decline in preventive services while enabling vulnerable adults to stay safe at home. Self-reported vital signs collected by patients may be used. The required elements of health risk assessment, review of functional ability and level of safety, review of past medical and family history, screen for cognitive impairment and depression, medication reconciliation, and list of current providers and DME suppliers can easily be conducted via live synchronous video connection. The visit concludes with preventive health education and counseling based on individual risk factors and referrals for screenings and community support, which can be accomplished via telemedicine. The written preventive screening checklist should be published on the patient's electronic portal or mailed after the visit.

Chronic Disease Management

Dementia

Telemedicine is more frequently used for neuropsychiatric care than other specialties and is effective for this application in geriatric patients. There is evidence that standardized tools like the Mini-Mental State Examination (MMSE) and Montreal Cognitive Assessment (MoCA) can reliably be administered in telehealth encounters (see **Table 1**).[24,25] A recent systematic review evaluating synchronous video visits suggested reliability similar to in-person visits.[24] These assessments may also be applied in other forms of telehealth, such as smartphone-based assessments, internet-based reminders and games, web-based educational programs, mobile text messaging, and chat forums.[26]

Dementia was one of the most common conditions using telehealth in a recent review of published articles during the COVID-19 pandemic.[3] Strengths of telehealth included the provision of holistic health care in the home and other remote settings while avoiding infection risk. Studies show telehealth is feasible and well-accepted in this setting; however, data on the cognitive effects of dementia care are limited with mixed results. Outcomes of telemedicine via audio-visual consultation for dementia in rural elderly patients were reported in a systematic review of 12 studies by Sekhon and colleagues.[27] All the studies were observational, with one comparing telemedicine to face-to-face visits. In this study, video consultation was provided by a dementia specialist with assistance from providers at a rural public health center.[28] The mean point decline in MMSE per year was not significantly different between groups (0.60 for telemedicine vs 1.03 for face-to-face visits), suggesting that telemedicine is an effective alternative to face-to-face visits for rural patients with dementia.

Depression

There are validated tools for the assessment of mental health status that can be used through telehealth, such as the Patient Health Questionnaire 2-item (PHQ-2) and the Geriatric Depression Scale (GDS).[4,24] One study in NH residents using video counseling once per week showed a significant difference in the GDS compared with standard NH care. In another randomized, noninferiority trial, Egede and colleagues[29] compared telemedicine to same-room treatment of major depressive disorder. The intervention was delivered by videophone in 8 weekly psychotherapy sessions in the veteran population. About 70% of the participants were rural residents. The criteria for noninferiority were met at 12 months of follow-up for the GDS with treatment response of 22% in the telemedicine group and 20% in the same-room treatment group. Similar results were seen for the Beck Depression Inventory (BDI) with responses of 24% and 23%, for telemedicine and same-room treatment, respectively.

Heart failure

In an open-label RCT, Comin-Colet and colleagues[30] evaluated a heart failure program with telemedicine in place of face-to-face visits. Patients assigned to telemedicine used automated home telemonitoring with virtual encounters. Biometric data and patient-reported symptoms were gathered through a Bluetooth-enabled tablet and sent to a clinical workstation. The mean age of patients was 74 years and 25% were considered frail. The primary endpoint was nonfatal heart failure events during 6 months of follow-up. The hazard ratio was 0.35 (95% CI, 0.20–0.59, $P < .001$) for telemedicine compared with face-to-face visits. In addition to reducing heart failure events, there was a reduction in readmissions in the telemedicine group with a decrease in costs. There was a high degree of acceptance and satisfaction with telemedicine.

Diabetes mellitus

In another randomized study of older adults (mean age 71 years) with diabetes, Trief and colleagues[31] compared telemedicine case management to usual care. The intervention consisted of video visits every 4 to 6 weeks with an educator to monitor progress and set goals to improve adherence to self-care. The outcome was measured using a questionnaire whereby higher scores indicated more days of adherence to diet, exercise, and blood glucose testing. During 5 years of follow-up, subjects in the telemedicine group had higher mean scores than usual care indicating better adherence ($P < .001$). Overall adherence was also a significant mediator of better glycemic control.

Hypertension

Remote patient monitoring has been evaluated in older adults with several chronic health conditions, including heart failure, diabetes, hypertension, and chronic obstructive pulmonary disease. Programs for heart failure and hypertension may be less costly than other programs.[32] Rifkin and colleagues[33] randomized 43 participants at a VA clinic (mean age 68 years) with uncontrolled hypertension and chronic kidney disease to telemonitoring or usual care for 6 months. The RPM technology used a Bluetooth-enabled blood pressure device linked to a home transmitter that sent data to a secure website. Blood pressure readings were reviewed by study providers who called participants if it was out of range. The change from baseline in blood pressure was not significantly different between the telemonitoring and usual care groups (systolic change −13 mm Hg vs −8.5 mm Hg, respectively and diastolic change −3.5 mm Hg vs −8 mm Hg, respectively). Nearly all participants reported they would continue to use the technology if it was available after the study.

Overcoming Barriers to Telemedicine Care

User-specific considerations

The application of telehealth may be limited by user-dependent factors. Older patients and caregivers may lack access to the technology required for telemedicine care. Also, this population may not have the interest or ability to operate the technology.[3] Interventions that are designed to be simple are associated with positive clinical outcomes.[30,33]

A focus group interview-based study revealed acceptance of technology by older people was related to several predictors, including perceived usefulness, effort expectancy, computer anxiety, perceived security, social influences, and facilitating conditions.[1] In most of the focus groups, the recommendation of the physician was reported to influence the patient's decision to use home telemedicine services. A recent systematic review identified lack of staff training and health care provider resistance to the system as barriers to patient uptake of home telehealth systems.[34] This suggests the provider's message to the patient and efforts to facilitate the use of telemedicine influence its adoption by older adults.

It may be more challenging to treat patients with cognitive impairment or sensory limitations like visual acuity issues or hearing loss via telemedicine.[2,3] Doraiswamy and colleagues suggest future efforts include the development of automatic speech analysis to diagnose and monitor dementia, and improved technology to accommodate cognitive or sensory impairment.

Technology-specific considerations

Telehealth care may be affected by technical difficulties inherent to any technology-based system. Adequate support personnel are necessary to maintain equipment and troubleshoot technical difficulties.[35] Various technological issues such as difficulty establishing connection, transmission failure, poor audio-video connection, and equipment failure have been reported.[2,3,8] Back-up processes should be developed to enable continued care in the event of equipment malfunction or audio-visual disconnection. Dedicating time to addressing patient technological concerns and barriers and directing them to resources within the community or health care system to strengthen digital literacy may improve telehealth services for older people.[3]

Patient privacy and security are a concern in the vulnerable elderly population. The virtual platform may present missed opportunities for identifying clues of elder abuse due to lack of privacy.[3] In an analysis of 9 studies of 975 patients, 4 studies reported physician concern about confidentiality in telemedicine, like perceiving patients or their caregivers were unable to speak openly on the platform.[2] Secure software must be used to prevent hacking.

There are limitations to the physical examination that can be performed via telemedicine.[2] Many physicians perceive this as a weakness of the virtual platform.[2,3] In a national survey, 71% of older adults also voiced concern that their health care provider would not be able to do a thorough examination.[36] Diagnostic clues that are usually detected by the traditional in-person examination, like the detection of cardiac arrhythmia by auscultation or a subtle mass on abdominal palpation, may be missed in the remote examination. Therefore, it is important to obtain consent from the patient, advise them of potential limitations, and set expectations at the start of the virtual visit.[37] Currently, data are limited in comparing the validity of the virtual examination with the traditional examination.[37] Dewar and colleagues[36] published a model for an adapted physical examination for virtual geriatric clinic encounters, using the basic components of inspection, palpation, percussion, and auscultation. The "laying of hands" by the clinician in the traditional bedside examination, which strengthens the therapeutic physician-patient connection, is lost in a remote telemedicine examination and may increase the risk of depersonalized care. These barriers can be overcome by using an in-person encounter for the initial consultation, with follow-up conducted virtually.[2]

A limitation to the virtual Medicare AWV is the inability to administer vaccinations or draw bloodwork at the point of care that are available in a typical office-based encounter, potentially leading to delays in preventive care. Research efforts should be directed toward gauging the long-term effects of delayed preventive health screenings during the pandemic on seniors, as well as the adoption and efficacy of the virtual AWV by providers.

Financial Impact and Reimbursement Policies

Health care costs

As the Baby Boomer generation ages, US health care expenditures continue to rise in response to more prevalent complex disease states.[38] Prior research has shown that telehealth can reduce health care costs and improve health outcomes through improvement in health metrics like hospital readmission rates, emergency department visits, glycosylated hemoglobin A1C, blood pressure, and heart failure morbidity and mortality.[39] In opposition to this, there is concern about telehealth being overutilized by patients and providers, and some evidence demonstrating higher downstream health care costs due to increased testing and follow up visits.[40] As the future of telemedicine continues to be debated, more research is needed to better inform providers, payers, and policy makers on the nuanced cost-effectiveness of telehealth patient care.[41]

New Medicare policies

The SARS-CoV-2 pandemic provided a catalyst for CMS to adopt both short-term and long-term telehealth policy changes for patients with Medicare. Policy changes temporarily permitted providers to bill for remote services for both new and established patients inside their homes, including across state lines. Initially, in 2020, the 3 main Medicare virtual services included audio-only and video telehealth visits, virtual check-ins, and e-visits.[42] Approximately 40% of primary care visits received by Medicare beneficiaries early in the pandemic were telemedicine visits, both audio-only and audio-video visits.[43]

Temporary versus permanent Centers for Medicare and Medicaid Services policy changes

As part of CMS policy changes for the 2021 Physician Fee Schedule (PFS), both temporary and permanent policy categories for telehealth services were created. Permanent "Category 1" virtual services include psychiatric care, simple remote home visits, and prolonged services. Temporary policies are "Category 3" virtual services reimbursed during the public health emergency (PHE) only, including complex remote

Table 2
Centers for Medicare and Medicaid Services (CMS) outpatient telehealth services

CPT Code	2021 CMS Payment	wRVU	Description
97802	$37.69	0.53	Medical nutrition, individual[a]
97804	$17.10	0.23	Medical nutrition, group[a]
99202–05	$73.97, $113.75, $169.93, $224.36	1.10, 1.51, 2.04, 2.62	Office/outpatient visit new[b]
99212–15	$56.88, $92.47, $131.20, $183.19	0.88, 1.25, 1.70, 2.80	Office/outpatient visit established[b]
99347–48	$54.78 $83.74	1.00 1.56	Home visit established patient[a]
99349–50	$129.10 $178.65	2.33 3.28	Home visit established patient[a] -*Available up to December 31st, 2023*
99406 99407	$15.70 $25.82	0.24 0.50	Behavioral change for smoking (3–10 min, >10 min)[a]
99495 99496	$207.96 $281.59	2.78 3.79	Transitional care management, moderate (<14 d) or high (<7 d s/p discharge)[b]
99497	$85.84	1.50	Advanced care planning[a]
G0438 G0439	$169.23 $133.64	2.60 1.92	Annual Wellness Visit (AWV), initial[a] Annual Wellness Visit (AWV), subsequent[a]
G0442 G0443	$18.84 $26.87	0.18 0.45	Annual alcohol screening[a] Brief alcohol misuse counselling[a]
G0444	$18.84	0.18	Annual depression screening[a]
G0446	$26.87	0.45	Intensive behavioral therapy, CV disease[a]
G0447	$26.87	0.45	Behavioral counseling for obesity[a]
G2252	$26.87	0.50	Brief patient check-in, 11–20 min[a]

[a] Audio-only is permitted, under certain circumstances.
[b] Requires both audio AND video technology.
Data from Refs.[44,51]

home visits, physical and occupational therapy, emergency department and hospital care, and NH care. Virtual NH visits were expanded so that providers could bill a visit every 14 days instead of every 30 days. Other virtual services added by CMS in 2021 included virtual Medicare AWV (initial or subsequent AWV, but not the Initial Preventive Physical Examination), cognitive impairment assessments, advance care planning, RPM, and transitional care management services (**Table 2**).[44]

Audio-only telemedicine
A new G code (G2252) introduced by CMS in the 2021 PFS covered audio-only assessments, which can be billed if greater than 5 to 10 minutes is required to determine the need for an in-person visit.[45] Of note, reimbursement for outpatient video follow-up visits and for audio-only follow-up visits were not included in the 2021 or 2022 CMS PFS changes. During the pandemic, audio-only telemedicine visits were temporarily reimbursed by CMS, given that some seniors lacked access to or experience with

video technology.[43] Current telehealth reimbursement policies often require video to be incorporated, as video visits are generally thought to provide better patient assessments and allow for better physician-patient communication using visual cues and rapport building. Audio-only encounters have been shown to take less time, although physician medical decision-making can be the same as with an in-person encounter.[43] Late in 2021 through advocacy efforts from the American Medical Association and other organized medicine groups, modifier 93 was adopted by the CPT (Current Procedural Terminology) Editorial Panel to allow reporting of audio-only synchronous telemedicine services. This modifier became effective on January 1st, 2022, although payment has yet to be determined.[46]

Extension of services added during the pandemic

As more is learned about the benefits and limitations of various telehealth services, CMS continues to revise the PFS. Certain services temporarily covered during the pandemic were extended for 2022 and 2023, permitting additional evaluation and data collection. When diagnosing and treating a mental health disorder, it is permissible for the originating site to be the patient's home, with a requirement of at least one in-person visit at least every 12 months.[47] Specific nursing facility, nutrition, and remote home visit services were added to permanent CMS telehealth services, as well as the initial and annual Medicare AWV and associated counseling services. New and established outpatient telemedicine visits continue to be reimbursed into 2022, requiring both audio and video. Of note, virtual home visits and outpatient telemedicine visits have different reimbursement amounts and requirements.[44]

Regulatory advocacy

To promote the Triple Aim in virtual geriatric care (improve quality of care, the patient experience, and reduce cost), it is imperative for all primary care providers to advocate for responsible and ethical virtual services.[5] Telehealth policies and procedures should be written to protect patient privacy, ensure equity and access for all patients, and define an expected level of patient care at or above generally accepted standards of in-person and virtual health care.[48] Providers should help revise telehealth licensure requirements, billing laws, and documentation guidelines. Telehealth policies should be regulated by the medical community and not by financially motivated stakeholders. Meaningful regulatory and health care policy changes are essential for ensuring appropriate and equitable telehealth care for our vulnerable aging patient population, driven by local and national health care provider advocacy efforts.[49]

SUMMARY

Telehealth provides an opportunity for expanded health care services for a growing geriatric population facing challenges related to health care. For older adults with limited transportation, it offers a way for patients, family, caregivers, and providers to communicate and coordinate care. Telehealth is a viable alternative to in-person care for common geriatric assessments by videoconferencing or medication reconciliation by telephone. Various forms of telehealth have been evaluated for health promotion and disease management, including mHealth, remote telemonitoring, online forums or portals, email, and text-messaging. Studies evaluating outcomes of telehealth in older adults have suggested benefits in many areas of care. However, there is variability in the design of studies and more RCTs are needed to establish benefits. Even so, data that are available support the feasibility of telehealth and patient satisfaction with this model of care. Telehealth interventions should be designed carefully to ensure usability and security. As the field of telehealth continues to evolve, it is imperative that both patients and providers advocate for national regulatory policies and reimbursement strategies promoting equitable, high-quality, and cost-effective geriatric telehealth models.

CLINICS CARE POINTS

- Clinicians should become comfortable using various telehealth interventions (including telemedicine encounters, RPM, and mobile health technologies) when caring for geriatric patients, ideally partnering with caregivers and other health care professionals when obstacles are identified.

- It is important for clinicians to familiarize themselves with evidence-based telemedicine geriatric assessment tools to optimize remote evaluation of geriatric patients.

- Having a simplified onboarding process, with both office-based and home-based support systems to enhance usability, will help older patients overcome barriers to telehealth.

- Clinicians should continually be aware of CMS telehealth policy changes, as reimbursement and regulatory policies will continue to change as more is learned about the field of telehealth.

- Promotion of responsible virtual geriatric care should be encouraged through local and regional advocacy efforts, focusing on the triple aim of health care (quality, patient experience, and cost).

DISCLOSURE

The authors have nothing to disclose.

REFERENCES

1. Cimperman M, Brenčič MM, Trkman P, et al. Older adults' perceptions of home telehealth services. Telemed J E Health 2013;19(10):786–90.
2. Murphy RP, Dennehy KA, Costello MM, et al. Virtual geriatric clinics and the COVID-19 catalyst: a rapid review. Age Ageing 2020;49(6):907–14.
3. Doraiswamy S, Jithesh A, Mamtani R, et al. Telehealth use in geriatrics care during the COVID-19 pandemic-a scoping review and evidence synthesis. Int J Environ Res Public Health 2021;18(4):1755.
4. DiGiovanni G, Mousaw K, Lloyd T, et al. Development of a telehealth geriatric assessment model in response to the COVID-19 pandemic. J Geriatr Oncol 2020;11(5):761–3.
5. Vockley M. The rise of telehealth: 'triple aim,' innovative technology, and popular demand are spearheading new models of health and wellness care. Biomed Instrum Technol 2015;49(5):306–20.
6. Frost R, Nimmons D, Davies N. Using remote interventions in promoting the health of frail older persons following the COVID-19 lockdown: challenges and solutions. J Am Med Dir Assoc 2020;21(7):992–3.
7. Sanford JA, Butterfield T. Using remote assessment to provide home modification services to underserved elders. Gerontologist 2005;45(3):389–98.
8. Gately ME, Trudeau SA, Moo LR. Feasibility of Telehealth-Delivered Home Safety Evaluations for Caregivers of Clients With Dementia. OTJR (Thorofare N J) 2020; 40(1):42–9.

9. Frank C, Godwin M, Verma S, et al. What drugs are our frail elderly patients taking? Do drugs they take or fail to take put them at increased risk of interactions and inappropriate medication use? Can Fam Physician 2001;47:1198–204.

10. Lavan AH, Gallagher PF, O'Mahony D. Methods to reduce prescribing errors in elderly patients with multimorbidity. Clin Interv Aging 2016;11:857–66.

11. Liu VC, Mohammad I, Deol BB, et al. Post-discharge medication reconciliation: reduction in readmissions in a geriatric primary care clinic. J Aging Health 2019;31(10):1790–805.

12. Paquin AM, Salow M, Rudolph JL. Pharmacist calls to older adults with cognitive difficulties after discharge in a Tertiary Veterans Administration Medical Center: a quality improvement program. J Am Geriatr Soc 2015;63(3):571–7.

13. Kane-Gill SL, Wong A, Culley CM, et al. Transforming the medication regimen review process using telemedicine to prevent adverse events. J Am Geriatr Soc 2021;69(2):530–8.

14. Yerrakalva D, Yerrakalva D, Hajna S, et al. Effects of mobile health app interventions on sedentary time, physical activity, and fitness in older adults: systematic review and meta-analysis. J Med Internet Res 2019;21(11):e14343.

15. Lyons EJ, Swartz MC, Lewis ZH, et al. Feasibility and acceptability of a wearable technology physical activity intervention with telephone counseling for mid-aged and older adults: a randomized controlled pilot trial. JMIR Mhealth Uhealth 2017; 5(3):e28.

16. Ashe MC, Winters M, Hoppmann CA, et al. "Not just another walking program": everyday activity supports you (EASY) model-a randomized pilot study for a parallel randomized controlled trial. Pilot Feasibility Stud 2015;1:4.

17. Nunez de Arenas-Arroyo S, Cavero-Redondo I, Alvarez-Bueno C, et al. Effect of eHealth to increase physical activity in healthy adults over 55 years: a systematic review and meta-analysis. Scand J Med Sci Sports 2021;31(4):776–89.

18. van Doorn-van Atten MN, Haveman-Nies A, van Bakel MM, et al. Effects of a multi-component nutritional telemonitoring intervention on nutritional status, diet quality, physical functioning and quality of life of community-dwelling older adults. Br J Nutr 2018;119(10):1185–94.

19. Marx W, Kelly JT, Crichton M, et al. Is telehealth effective in managing malnutrition in community-dwelling older adults? A systematic review and meta-analysis. Maturitas 2018;111:31–46.

20. (CMS) CfMaMS. Medicare wellness visits. centers for medicare and medicaid services. 2021. Available at: https://www.cms.gov/Outreach-and-Education/Medicare-Learning-Network-MLN/MLNProducts/preventive-services/medicare-wellness-visits.html. Accessed October 15, 2021.

21. Daily D. How COVID-19 made the annual wellness visit more important than ever. prevounce blog. Available at: https://blog.prevounce.com/how-covid-19-made-the-annual-wellness-visit-more-important-than-ever. Accessed October 25, 2021.

22. Gorin SNS, Jimbo M, Heizelman R, et al. The future of cancer screening after COVID-19 may be at home. Cancer 2021;127(4):498–503.

23. El Khoury C, Haro E, Alves M, et al. Patient-centered home cancer screening attitudes during COVID-19 pandemic. J Patient Cent Res Rev 2021;8(4):340–6.

24. Gentry MT, Lapid MI, Rummans TA. Geriatric Telepsychiatry: Systematic Review and Policy Considerations. Am J Geriatr Psychiatry 2019;27(2):109–27.

25. Nasreddine Z. Remote MoCA testing. Available at: https://www.mocatest.org/faq/. Accessed November 30, 2021.

26. Cuffaro L, Di Lorenzo F, Bonavita S, et al. Dementia care and COVID-19 pandemic: a necessary digital revolution. Neurol Sci 2020;41(8):1977–9.

27. Sekhon H, Sekhon K, Launay C, et al. Telemedicine and the rural dementia population: a systematic review. Maturitas 2021;143:105–14.
28. Kim H, Jhoo JH, Jang JW. The effect of telemedicine on cognitive decline in patients with dementia. J Telemed Telecare 2017;23(1):149–54.
29. Egede LE, Acierno R, Knapp RG, et al. Psychotherapy for depression in older veterans via telemedicine: a randomised, open-label, non-inferiority trial. Lancet Psychiatry 2015;2(8):693–701.
30. Comin-Colet J, Enjuanes C, Verdu-Rotellar JM, et al. Impact on clinical events and healthcare costs of adding telemedicine to multidisciplinary disease management programmes for heart failure: Results of a randomized controlled trial. J Telemed Telecare 2016;22(5):282–95.
31. Trief PM, Izquierdo R, Eimicke JP, et al. Adherence to diabetes self care for white, African-American and Hispanic American telemedicine participants: 5 year results from the IDEATel project. Ethn Health 2013;18(1):83–96.
32. Peretz D, Arnaert A, Ponzoni NN. Determining the cost of implementing and operating a remote patient monitoring programme for the elderly with chronic conditions: A systematic review of economic evaluations. J Telemed Telecare 2018; 24(1):13–21.
33. Rifkin DE, Abdelmalek JA, Miracle CM, et al. Linking clinic and home: a randomized, controlled clinical effectiveness trial of real-time, wireless blood pressure monitoring for older patients with kidney disease and hypertension. Blood Press Monit 2013;18(1):8–15.
34. Almathami HKY, Win KT, Vlahu-Gjorgievska E. Barriers and facilitators that influence telemedicine-based, real-time, online consultation at patients' homes: systematic literature review. J Med Internet Res 2020;22(2):e16407.
35. Shafiee Hanjani L, Bell JS, Freeman C. Undertaking medication review by telehealth. Aust J Gen Pract 2020;49(12):826–31.
36. Dewar S, Lee PG, Suh TT, et al. Uptake of virtual visits in a geriatric primary care clinic during the COVID-19 pandemic. J Am Geriatr Soc 2020;68(7):1392–4.
37. Ansary AM, Martinez JN, Scott JD. The virtual physical exam in the 21st century. J Telemed Telecare 2021;27(6):382–92.
38. Kampmeijer R, Pavlova M, Tambor M, et al. The use of e-health and m-health tools in health promotion and primary prevention among older adults: a systematic literature review. BMC Health Serv Res 2016;16(Suppl 5):290.
39. Mahtta D, Daher M, Lee MT, et al. Promise and perils of telehealth in the current era. Curr Cardiol Rep 2021;23(9):115.
40. Ashwood JS, Mehrotra A, Cowling D, et al. Direct-to-consumer telehealth may increase access to care but does not decrease spending. Health Aff (Millwood) 2017;36(3):485–91.
41. Eze ND, Mateus C, Cravo Oliveira Hashiguchi T. Telemedicine in the OECD: An umbrella review of clinical and cost-effectiveness, patient experience and implementation. PLoS One 2020;15(8):e0237585.
42. (CMS) CfMaMS. Medicare telemedicine healthcare provider fact Sheet. Available at: https://www.cms.gov/newsroom/fact-sheets/medicare-telemedicine-healthcare-provider-fact-sheet. Accessed January 1, 2022.
43. Benjenk I, Franzini L, Roby D, et al. Disparities in audio-only telemedicine use among medicare beneficiaries during the coronavirus disease 2019 pandemic. Med Care 2021;59(11):1014–22.
44. (CMS) CfMaMS. List of Telehealth Services for Calendar Year. 2022. Available at: https://www.cms.gov/Medicare/Medicare-General-Information/Telehealth/Telehealth-Codes. Accessed January 1, 2022.

45. (CMS) CfMaMS. Final Policy, Payment, and Quality Provisions Changes to the Medicare Physician Fee Schedule for Calendar Year. 2021. Available at: https://www.cms.gov/newsroom/fact-sheets/final-policy-payment-and-quality-provisions-changes-medicare-physician-fee-schedule-calendar-year-1. Accessed January 1, 2022.

46. CPT® Appendix A audio only Modifier 93 for reporting medical services. 2022. Available at: https://www.ama-assn.org/practice-management/cpt/cpt-appendix-audio-only-modifier-93-reporting-medical-services. Accessed January 6, 2022.

47. (CMS) CfMaMS. CMS Newsroom, Calendar Year (CY) 2022 Medicare Physician Fee Schedule Final Rule. Available at: https://www.cms.gov/newsroom/fact-sheets/calendar-year-cy-2022-medicare-physician-fee-schedule-final-rule. Accessed January 1, 2022.

48. Romani PW, Schieltz KM. Ethical Considerations When Delivering Behavior Analytic Services for Problem Behavior via Telehealth. Behav Anal (Wash D C) 2017; 17(4):312–24.

49. North S. These Four Telehealth Changes Should Stay, Even After the Pandemic. Fam Pract Manag 2021;28(3):9–11.

50. Chang W, Homer M, Rossi MI. Use of clinical video telehealth as a tool for optimizing medications for rural older veterans with dementia. Geriatrics (Basel) 2018;3(3):44.

51. (CMS) CfMaMS. Medicare Physician Fee Schedule Search Tool. Available at: https://www.cms.gov/medicare/physician-fee-schedule/search. Accessed January 1, 2022.

Urgent Care Through Telehealth

Eric W. Bean, DO, MBA[a], Kathryn M. Harmes, MD, MHSA[b],*

KEYWORDS

- Urgent care • Telehealth • Direct-to-consumer

KEY POINTS

- Urgent care has become a convenient, accessible alternative between primary and emergency care.
- Care for urgent conditions via telehealth has expanded since the COVID-19 pandemic.
- Direct-to-consumer companies provide access to on-demand, urgent telehealth care with mixed evidence regarding quality and utilization costs.

INTRODUCTION

Telehealth and urgent care are rapidly becoming essential sectors within the health care industry. The COVID-19 pandemic has accelerated the use of telehealth as patients seek safe, reliable access to acute care while minimizing risks of exposure. Current health care trends and patient preferences have convened to bring these 2 health care modalities together in the form of urgent care telehealth (UCT). This article explores the history of telehealth and urgent care individually, then examines their intersection in UCT.

The authors focus on the benefits and the barriers to providing urgent care virtually and discuss quality and the costs of offering such services. These topics will provide the groundwork for predicting the future of UCT and its possible applications to meet patient needs.

THE GENESIS OF FAST CARE

Facilities offering walk-in care, initially staffed by entrepreneurial physicians, were opened in the 1970s to bypass the long waits found in hospital emergency

Neither author has conflicts of interest to disclose.

[a] Department of Emergency and Hospital Medicine, Lehigh Valley Health Network, 707 Hamilton Street, 5th Floor, Allentown, PA 18101, USA; [b] Department of Family Medicine, University of Michigan Medical School, 300 North Ingalls Street, NI4C06, Ann Arbor, MI 48109-5435, USA

* Corresponding author.

E-mail address: jordankm@umich.edu

primarycare.theclinics.com

departments (EDs). These early facilities eventually grew to a point where hospital systems saw losses in revenue and started offering similar services—and some would argue a higher quality of care—in the 1980s. As the number of sites increased, so did their offering of diagnostic services and simple procedures. In addition to convenience, their popularity was driven by the gaps in access to primary care and the high cost of emergency care.[1]

Urgent care centers by the current definition provide care primarily on a walk-in basis, are open evenings Monday through Friday and at least 1 day over the weekend, provide suturing for minor lacerations, and provide onsite radiographs.[2] Reimbursement rates, payer distribution, and physician salaries align more with office-based primary care than EDs. A 2018 study in *JAMA Internal Medicine* demonstrated a substantial shift in venues of care for patients with low-acuity conditions. Use of urgent care centers increased 138% from 2008 to 2015, whereas ED utilization decreased by 14%.[3] Although urgent care visits are less costly than the ED for comparable low-acuity care,[2] there is some evidence that wide availability of urgent care centers may raise overall net spending on health care owing to increased utilization.[4]

PATIENT PREFERENCES FOR DISTANCE HEALING

Before the COVID-19 pandemic, telehealth was slowly gaining traction worldwide. Data from the American Medical Association's 2016 Physician Practice Benchmark Survey demonstrated that 15.4% of physicians used telehealth for patient interactions. Utilization varied by specialty as well as practice size, with larger practices more likely to use the technology.[5] The COVID-19 pandemic served as a catalyst for significant expansion of telehealth. According to a 2020 *MMWR* report, telehealth encounters in March of 2020 increased by 154% ($P<.05$) compared with the same week in 2019.[6] Virtual urgent care (VUC) services also rapidly expanded during this time. A study of VUC at a New York health system demonstrated a 33-fold increase in visits from March-April 2019 to 2020.[7]

A 2020 online survey of more than 200 adults and 600 physicians demonstrated that 59% of patients had their first video visit during COVID-19.[8] Patients reported a willingness to participate in online care owing to time savings/convenience (58%), faster service (47%), cost savings (38%), safety concerns during COVID-19 (31%), and better access to health care professionals (26%). Of patients, 35% expressed willingness to use telehealth for urgent care complaints, whereas 53% of physicians expressed willingness to provide this care.

Preferences for video versus in-person visits were investigated using a sample of adult members of the RAND American Life Panel in March 2021.[9] Two thousand eighty patients were surveyed, with a mean age of 51.1 years. Of participants, 66.5% favored video visits in general, but more than half of respondents (53.0%) preferred in-person care when faced with a choice between modalities when cost was not a factor. When confronted with higher costs for in-person care, that number dropped to 49.8%.

A 2017 study by Welch and colleagues[10] surveyed 4345 respondents nationwide about willingness and comfort with telehealth. Of respondents, 52% were willing to see their own primary care provider (PCP) via telehealth; 35% were willing to see another provider from the same organization, and 19% were willing to see a different provider from another organization. These results support the provision of telehealth acute care from the medical home when access is available.

Smartphones are now found in 85% of Americans' pockets, according to Pew research in April 2021.[11] Patients now have near-immediate access to a telehealth evaluation. Preferences for virtual versus in-person care vary by age, with signs indicating that Millennials and Generation Z population prefer telehealth to traditional medicine.[8] As the pandemic eases, there are no signs of these distanced-care interactions decreasing, and there is a consensus that the utilization of telehealth in urgent care will continue to grow. The telehealth platform is on track to becoming an established tool for management of urgent care conditions.

A NEW MODEL OF ACUTE-VISIT CARE TAKES HOLD

Many patients have access to telehealth for acute care from their established physician or health system using functionality build into existing electronic medical record systems (EMRs). Direct-to-consumer (DTC) care has emerged as an alternative businesses model that offers access to online acute care in all 50 states. Teladoc, Amwell, and MDLive are examples of platforms offering on-demand acute care services.

To initiate a telemedicine visit through a DTC company like Teledoc or a local health networks' EMR such as EPIC, patients need to first download the application they will be using. Once the application is launched, the patient will be asked to agree with the conditions of service, which include an explanation of the service and legal considerations. Patients with emergent complaints necessitating a higher level of care, including but not limited to chest pain, stroke symptoms, and seizures, will be excluded and encouraged to seek emergent care elsewhere. If no exclusions apply, information on demographics, insurance coverage, and payment information is typically solicited. Patients will then choose their chief complaint from a list presented (**Table 1**).

In Teledoc and AmWell, for instance, before the start of the visit, the patient can see the provider's picture, education, and ratings. Patients can select the provider with whom they feel most comfortable based on the information provided. The patient is then placed in a queue and given an estimate of the wait time. Some services offer appointments for those who prefer not to wait.

Once the appointment ends, the patient is sent a digital copy of an after-visit summary. When needed, prescriptions are electronically prescribed. The patient is often sent a survey to elicit feedback after the encounter.

BENEFITS ON BOTH SIDES OF THE SCREEN

Convenience is a primary benefit to patients. Barriers to patient access to in-person care can include, but are not limited to, transportation issues, childcare concerns, and coordination of schedules to match appointment availability. There is also a time cost to transportation to and from the office, parking logistics, registration, and in-person triage. These barriers could all be eliminated with the use of UCT. Time is decreased to just a few minutes on an app before being seen. Subsequent usage can be more efficient if demographic and insurance information is stored on the application.

Table 1
Common conditions that could be managed by telehealth

• Urinary problems	• Pink eye
• Ear pain	• Cough/cold symptoms
• Rashes	• COVID-19 symptoms and exposure
• Allergies	• Back pain
• Nausea	• Medication questions and refill requests
• Insect bites	
• Follow-up visits	

There are large upfront expenses in opening an urgent-care center, which include staffing, marketing, and other initial operating expenses. A UCT virtual presence minimizes some of these barriers to entry into a market. The ability to scale based on demand is much greater with UCT, as providers work remotely.

A 2018 to 2019 survey of DTC UCT providers identified many facilitators.[12] Workplace factors, including reliable technology with real-time IT support and easy access to EHR for patient records, were found to be supportive of high-quality care. Experience in in-person care was also thought to be essential. Active listening skills and attention to nonverbal cues were thought to contribute to accurate diagnoses. In addition, clinicians identified the need to exhibit confidence in communication and diagnoses.

BARRIERS TO URGENT-CARE TELEMEDICINE

Despite the many benefits of using telehealth in the urgent-care setting, the platform does have some barriers to further adoption and expansion. Even with the best connectivity and image quality, there are limits to the ability to conduct a physical examination. Other barriers involve licensing, payment parity, uncertainty of regulatory or legislative changes post-COVID-19, and perception of value.

State licensure regulations have not kept pace with telemedicine. Licensure, granted and regulated at the state level, is based on the location of the patient, not that of the clinician. DTC providers require licensing in multiple states. The one exception to these limits in offering telehealth across states is the Veterans Administration, which grants its providers reciprocity in all 50 states.

Before the COVID-19 pandemic, much of telehealth was limited because of payment challenges and variability in state-to-state regulations. Some states required payment parity, and others did not require insurance to cover any telemedicine services. During the public health emergency due to the COVID-19 pandemic, the Centers for Medicare and Medicaid Services (CMS) enacted waivers to allow for services to be covered with payment parity. It is uncertain whether these waivers will continue postpandemic. It is thought that telehealth services will continue to be covered, but which services and to what extent are still to be determined.

Although most clinicians agree a good patient health history is key to diagnosing a current condition, a supporting examination is often helpful in making a final diagnosis. Despite a smartphone's capabilities, the ability to perform an otoscope examination, to listen to heart and lung sounds, and to perform a tactile/palpation examination is not possible. For these reasons, the conditions amenable to UCT may be limited.

Some may feel that telemedicine can weaken the doctor-patient relationship, and that it should not replace face-to-face care. The study of DTC providers found that mismatched expectations between patients and clinicians could result in added tension during the encounter.[12] Doing the right thing clinically for the health of the patient does not always meet the patient's expectations.

QUALITY OF URGENT-CARE TELEMEDICINE

An *Annals of Internal Medicine* 2021 study reviewed 38 randomized control trials and concluded that video teleconferencing resulted in similar clinical effectiveness, health care use, patient satisfaction, and quality of life when compared with usual care across many applications.[13] Current evidence is mixed as to the quality of UTC versus usual care, with many studies raising concern about antibiotic overuse in DTC practice.

A 2016 study compared quality of care at a DTC company with that at physicians' offices for patients enrolled in the California Public Employees' Retirement System HMO.[14] DTC providers were less likely to order recommended diagnostic testing for pharyngitis complaints (3% vs 50%) than providers at physician offices (P<.01). They were also less likely to avoid antibiotic prescription for bronchitis (16.7% vs 27.9; P<.01). Comparable performance was noted on back pain measures, with 88% versus 79% of providers not ordering imaging (P = .02).

A 2019 study compared DTC telehealth to in-person urgent care and PCP visits for pediatric acute respiratory infections.[15] Antibiotic prescribing was higher for DTC telemedicine visits (52%) compared with 42% of urgent care and 31% of PCP visits (P<.001 for both comparisons). Care concordant with guidelines for antibiotic use was lower with DTC visits (59%) compared with 67% of urgent care and 78% of PCP visits (P<.001). It should be noted that the American Academy of Pediatrics has discouraged the use of acute care services outside of the Medical Home owing to concerns for quality and continuity of care.[16]

A higher rate of antibiotic use for acute respiratory infection through DTC care was also demonstrated in a retrospective analysis of care provided to health system employees and dependents at a large urban academic health system.[17] Of 257 telehealth visits reviewed, patients seen by DTC providers had 2.3 higher odds of being prescribed antibiotics compared with system-affiliated physicians (95% confidence interval [CI], 1.1–4.5; P<.01).

Patient expectation may be influencing prescription patterns. A group from the Cleveland Clinic analyzed 8437 DTC encounters for respiratory tract infections and found that 66.1% resulted in prescription of an antibiotic; 15.5.% resulted in prescription of a nonantibiotic medication, and 18.3% resulted in no prescriptions.[18] Of those patients who received an antibiotic prescription, 90.9% rated their satisfaction with the interaction as 5 stars, compared with 72.5% of those who received no prescription and 86.0% of those who received a prescription for a nonantibiotic medication. Providers who prescribed antibiotics were more likely to receive a 5-star rating (odds ratio [OR], 3.23; 95% CI, 1.80–2.71) than those who did not provide any prescription.

When telehealth for low-acuity, urgent conditions is provided within an integrated health network where treatment protocols are applied consistently, the quality of care provided may be less variable. A 2021 study of claims from Intermountain Healthcare Network evaluated 182,853 claims across virtual care, urgent care, PCP, and ED settings.[19] There were no differences in rates of follow-up or antibiotic use between care settings. This was thought to be due to strict use of evidence-based care process models designed to maintain antibiotic stewardship.

UTILIZATION AND COST-EFFECTIVENESS OF URGENT CARE TELEHEALTH

Telehealth tends to be less expensive per visit than ED or in-person urgent care. A 2017 study of claims from a large commercial health insurer estimated that care from retail health clinics, urgent care centers, EDs, or PCP for acute, nonurgent conditions were $36, $153, $1735, and $162 per episode more expensive than virtual visits, respectively.[20]

Concern has been raised that the expanded access and availability of visits may be associated with increased overall health care spending. A 2017 study reviewed commercial claims data on more than 300,000 patients over 3 years for acute respiratory visits.[21] It was estimated that 12% of DTC telehealth visits replaced visits to other providers, whereas 88% of visits represented new utilization. Net spending on acute respiratory illness increased by $45 per telehealth user.

A subsequent prospective observational study of 650 patient encounters included direct patient surveys about alternatives to telemedicine visit.[22] Of these patients, 74% had their concerns resolved on the telemedicine visit without subsequent need for follow-up. Only 16% reported that they would have "done nothing" if the telehealth visit were not available. This is a much lower estimated rate of new utilization than shown previously. Using cost data, the researchers estimated a net cost savings of $19 to $121 per telehealth visit.

The Intermountain Healthcare study demonstrated significant cost savings for virtual care compared with PCP visits (−$278), urgent care (−$232), and ED (−$2974).[20] Jefferson Healthcare System's on-demand telehealth platform also demonstrated a $19 to $121 savings per telehealth visit to the patient.[22]

IMPLICATIONS FOR HEALTH EQUITY

Theoretically, UCT could improve access to care for patients in rural or urban underserved areas. It is unclear thus far whether UCT has proven to reduce health equity across populations. The 2016 study of DTC users demonstrated that patients were not more likely to be located within a health care professional shortage area (OR, 1.12) or rural location (OR, 1.0).[14] The 2020 consumer survey indicated that consumers in rural areas were less likely to have used telehealth (15%) than those in urban areas (25%) and suburban areas (23%).[8] Availability of broadband service may be one reason for this disparity.

A recent study of the Rochester, New York area population compared utilization for acute illness in children with and without telemedicine access, from 1993 to 2007.[23] The rates of acute visits before telemedicine were 75% greater among suburban children than inner-city children (OR, 1.75; P<.0001). When telemedicine became available to inner-city children, their overall active visits reached those of suburban children (OR, 0.80; P = .07). Researchers concluded that telehealth had the potential to redress socioeconomic disparities in acute care access.

HOW IT WILL LOOK: URGENT CARE TELEHEALTH'S PROBABLE FUTURE

Patients will continue to demand access and engage in their health care in ways that are easier and less expensive than other available options. For UCT to grow, it will need to address some of the barriers that limit a comprehensive physical examination, EMR integration, referrals for follow-up when appropriate, and triage to in-person care sites when needed.

Remote patient monitoring tools, such as digital scales, blood pressure monitors, glucometers, and pulse oximeters, are likely to become more available to patients. Bluetooth peripheral devices that give providers the capability to auscultate the heart, lung, and abdominal sounds in UCT interactions can expand on the physical examination. Camera attachments can allow providers look in the ears and nose to diagnose otitis media and sinus disease.

Point-of-care testing is becoming much more common as well. Glucometers, rapid COVID-19 tests, urine dipstick testing, and drug testing are all available now at the local pharmacy. There are companies that are looking to expand the conditions for which they can provide testing. In many cases, the results are digitally sent to your phone and can be integrated into the provider's EMR.

Integration of EMR will also continue to be important for accuracy of provider diagnosis and for patient reassurance that their care is comprehensive and coordinated. UCT that has access to the patient's records allows for a more detailed past medical history, current medications, previous office/virtual visits, and any testing that may have been done.

UCT may not be able to fully evaluate and treat a patient, and the patient may need to be directed to an ED or urgent-care center. Coordination of care and communication will facilitate care for the patient. Having dedicated referral patterns and agreements with in-person sites will help smooth this process.

CASE STUDY

A patient develops burning, frequency, and urgency of urination consistent with UTI. She is currently on vacation and unable to find a local urgent care, so she uses the DTC online health care service that has contracted with her insurance provider. She completes the visit and receives a prescription for a fluoroquinolone, which is sent to a local pharmacy. The patient experiences relief of her symptoms with treatment and enjoys the rest of her vacation.

Shortly after returning home, the patient starts to experience abdominal cramping and loose stools. She contacts her PCP, who is available for a same-day urgent visit via video. The PCP reviews her past medical history that includes a previous episode of *Clostridioides difficile* colitis precipitated by the same antibiotic she took while on vacation. The PCP orders stool studies to confirm reinfection, treats with oral metronidazole, and follows the patient's course of illness to resolution. She educates the patient to be cautious about treatment with broad-spectrum antibiotics in the future.

SUMMARY

As health care costs continue to increase, access challenges persist, and patient needs and expectations shift, UCT will continue to be an integral part of the health care system.

Urgent care will continue to fill the void between primary care and the ED setting, and it is likely that urgent care will evolve to consistently include UCT. To move this evolution forward, CMS waivers will need to become permanent. Telehealth should be reimbursed in accordance with in-person care. Constant advancements in technology will enhance examination capabilities, which will increase the conditions that can be treated virtually. When coupled with home testing, UCT could complement current models of health care and find its place as an integral part of every medical system and practice.

CLINICS CARE POINTS

- Urgent care telehealth can provide convenient access to health care for patients with urgent conditions.
- Urgent care telehealth services should be offered from the Patient Centered Medical Home (PCMH) to allow for continuity of care.
- Direct-to-consumer services are widely available and offered by many insurance plans.
- Antibiotic overuse is a concern, but may be avoided by use of standard, consistent guidelines.
- Urgent care telehealth has the potential to reduce utilization costs compared with emergency department and urgent cares, but increased convenience of care may create new utilization.
- Urgent care telehealth may improve health equity, provided areas have access to broadband Internet.

REFERENCES

1. McNeeley, S. Urgent Care Centers: An Overview. Am J Clinic Med: Vol 9, No. 2, 80-81.
2. Weinick RM, Bristol SJ, DesRoches CM. Urgent care centers in the U.S.: findings from a national survey. BMC Health Serv Res 2009;9:79.
3. Poon SJ, Schuur JD, Mehrotra A. Trends in Visits to Acute Care Venues for Treatment of Low-Acuity Conditions in the United States From 2008 to 2015. JAMA Intern Med 2018;178(10):1342–9.
4. Wang B, Mehrotra A, Friedman A. Urgent Care Centers Deter Some Emergency Department Visits But on Net, Increase Spending. Health Aff 2021;40(4):587–95.
5. Kane CK, Gillis K. The Use Of Telemedicine By Physicians: Still The Exception Rather Than The Rule. Health Aff (Millwood) 2018;37(12):1923–30.
6. Koonin LM, Hoots B, Tsang CA, et al. Trends in the use of telehealth during the emergency of the COVID-19 pandemic—United States, January–March 2020. MMWR Morb Mortal Wkly Rep 2020;69:1595–9.
7. Smith SW, Tiu J, Caspers CG, et al. Virtual Urgent Care Quality and Safety in the Time of Coronavirus. Jt Comm J Qual Patient Saf 2021;47(2):86–98.
8. Amwell. From virtual care to hybrid care: COVID-19 and the future of telehealth. Insights from the 2020 Amwell Physician and Consumer Survey. Available at: https://static.americanwell.com/app/uploads/2020/09/Amwell-2020-Physician-and-Consumer-Survey. pdf. Accessed March 13, 2022.
9. Predmore ZS, Roth E, Breslau J, et al. Assessment of Patient Preferences for Telehealth in Post-COVID-19 Pandemic Health Care. JAMA Netw Open 2021;4(12): e2136405.
10. Welch BM, Harvey J, O'Connell NS, et al. Patient preferences for direct-to-consumer telemedicine services: a nationwide survey. BMC Health Serv Res 2017;17(1):784.
11. Pew Research Center Feature. Mobile Fact Sheet. April 7, 2021. Available at: https://www.pewresearch.org/internet/fact-sheet/mobile/. Accessed January 23, 2022.
12. Laub N, Agarwal AK, Shi C, et al. Delivering Urgent Care Using Telemedicine: Insights from Experienced Clinicians at Academic Medical Centers. J Gen Intern Med 2022;37(4):707–13.
13. Albritton J, Ortiz A, Wines R, et al. Video Teleconferencing for Disease Prevention, Diagnosis, and Treatment : A Rapid Review. Ann Intern Med 2022;175(2):256–66.
14. Uscher-Pines L, Mulcahy A, Cowling D, et al. Access and Quality of Care in Direct-to-Consumer Telemedicine. Telemed J E Health 2016;22(4):282–7.
15. Ray KN, Shi Z, Gidengil CA, et al. Antibiotic Prescribing During Pediatric Direct-to-Consumer Telemedicine Visits. Pediatrics 2019;143(5):e20182491.
16. Conners GP, Kressly SJ, Perrin JM, et al, Committee on Practice and Ambulatory Medicine; Committee on Pediatric Emergency Medicine; Section on Telehealth Care; Section on Emergency Medicine; Subcommittee on Urgent Care; Task Force on Pediatric Practice Change. Nonemergency acute care: when it's not the medical home. Pediatrics 2017;139(5):e20170629.
17. Li KY, Ngai KM, Genes N. Differences in antibiotic prescribing rates for telemedicine encounters for acute respiratory infections. J Telemed Telecare 2022. https://doi.org/10.1177/1357633X221074503. 1357633X221074503.
18. Martinez KA, Rood M, Jhangiani N, et al. Association Between Antibiotic Prescribing for Respiratory Tract Infections and Patient Satisfaction in Direct-to-Consumer Telemedicine. JAMA Intern Med 2018;178(11):1558–60.

19. Lovell T, Albritton J, Dalto J, et al. Virtual vs traditional care settings for low-acuity urgent conditions: An economic analysis of cost and utilization using claims data. J Telemed Telecare 2021;27(1):59–65.
20. Gordon AS, Adamson WC, DeVries AR. Virtual Visits for Acute, Nonurgent Care: A Claims Analysis of Episode-Level Utilization. J Med Internet Res 2017; 19(2):e35.
21. Ashwood JS, Mehrotra A, Cowling D, et al. Direct-To-Consumer Telehealth May Increase Access To Care But Does Not Decrease Spending. Health Aff (Millwood) 2017;36(3):485–91.
22. Nord G, Rising KL, Band RA, et al. On-demand synchronous audio video telemedicine visits are cost effective. Am J Emerg Med 2019;37(5):890–4.
23. Ronis SD, McConnochie KM, Wang H, et al. Urban Telemedicine Enables Equity in Access to Acute Illness Care. Telemed J E Health 2017;23(2):105–12.

Statement of Ownership, Management, and Circulation
UNITED STATES POSTAL SERVICE® (All Periodicals Publications Except Requester Publications)

1. Publication Title
PRIMARY CARE: CLINICS IN OFFICE PRACTICE

2. Publication Number
044 – 690

3. Filing Date
9/18/2022

4. Issue Frequency
MAR, JUN, SEP, DEC

5. Number of Issues Published Annually
4

6. Annual Subscription Price
$269.00

7. Complete Mailing Address of Known Office of Publication (Not printer) (Street, city, county, state, and ZIP+4®)
ELSEVIER INC.
230 Park Avenue, Suite 800
New York, NY 10169

Contact Person
Malathi Samayan
Telephone (Include area code)
91-44-4299-4507

8. Complete Mailing Address of Headquarters or General Business Office of Publisher (Not printer)
ELSEVIER INC.
230 Park Avenue, Suite 800
New York, NY 10169

9. Full Names and Complete Mailing Addresses of Publisher, Editor, and Managing Editor (Do not leave blank)
Publisher (Name and complete mailing address)
Dolores Meloni, ELSEVIER INC.
1600 JOHN F KENNEDY BLVD. SUITE 1800
PHILADELPHIA, PA 19103-2899

Editor (Name and complete mailing address)
KATERINA HEIDHAUSEN, ELSEVIER INC.
1600 JOHN F KENNEDY BLVD. SUITE 1800
PHILADELPHIA, PA 19103-2899

Managing Editor (Name and complete mailing address)
PATRICK MANLEY, ELSEVIER INC.
1600 JOHN F KENNEDY BLVD. SUITE 1800
PHILADELPHIA, PA 19103-2899

10. Owner (Do not leave blank. If the publication is owned by a corporation, give the name and address of the corporation immediately followed by the names and addresses of all stockholders owning or holding 1 percent or more of the total amount of stock. If not owned by a corporation, give the names and addresses of the individual owners. If owned by a partnership or other unincorporated firm, give its name and address as well as those of each individual owner. If the publication is published by a nonprofit organization, give its name and address.)

Full Name	Complete Mailing Address
WHOLLY OWNED SUBSIDARY OF REED/ELSEVIER, US HOLDINGS	1600 JOHN F KENNEDY BLVD. SUITE 1800 PHILADELPHIA, PA 19103-2899

11. Known Bondholders, Mortgagees, and Other Security Holders Owning or Holding 1 Percent or More of Total Amount of Bonds, Mortgages, or Other Securities. If none, check box ▶ ☐ None

Full Name	Complete Mailing Address
N/A	

12. Tax Status (For completion by nonprofit organizations authorized to mail at nonprofit rates) (Check one)
The purpose, function, and nonprofit status of this organization and the exempt status for federal income tax purposes:
☒ Has Not Changed During Preceding 12 Months
☐ Has Changed During Preceding 12 Months (Publisher must submit explanation of change with this statement)

PS Form **3526**, July 2014 [Page 1 of 4 (see instructions page 4)] PSN: 7530-01-000-9931 PRIVACY NOTICE: See our privacy policy on www.usps.com.

13. Publication Title
PRIMARY CARE: CLINICS IN OFFICE PRACTICE

14. Issue Date for Circulation Data Below
JULY 2022

15. Extent and Nature of Circulation

			Average No. Copies Each Issue During Preceding 12 Months	No. Copies of Single Issue Published Nearest to Filing Date
a. Total Number of Copies (Net press run)			88	67
b. Paid Circulation (By Mail and Outside the Mail)	(1)	Mailed Outside-County Paid Subscriptions Stated on PS Form 3541 (include paid distribution above nominal rate, advertiser's proof copies, and exchange copies)	42	35
	(2)	Mailed In-County Paid Subscriptions Stated on PS Form 3541 (include paid distribution above nominal rate, advertiser's proof copies, and exchange copies)	0	0
	(3)	Paid Distribution Outside the Mails Including Sales Through Dealers and Carriers, Street Vendors, Counter Sales, and Other Paid Distribution Outside USPS®	14	8
	(4)	Paid Distribution by Other Classes of Mail Through the USPS (e.g., First-Class Mail®)	0	0
c. Total Paid Distribution (Sum of 15b (1), (2), (3), and (4))		▶	56	43
d. Free or Nominal Rate Distribution (By Mail and Outside the Mail)	(1)	Free or Nominal Rate Outside-County Copies included on PS Form 3541	16	7
	(2)	Free or Nominal Rate In-County Copies Included on PS Form 3541	0	0
	(3)	Free or Nominal Rate Copies Mailed at Other Classes Through the USPS (e.g., First-Class Mail)	0	0
	(4)	Free or Nominal Rate Distribution Outside the Mail (Carriers or other means)	0	0
e. Total Free or Nominal Rate Distribution (Sum of 15d (1), (2), (3) and (4))		▶	16	7
f. Total Distribution (Sum of 15c and 15e)		▶	72	50
g. Copies not Distributed (See instructions to Publishers #4 (page #3))		▶	16	17
h. Total (Sum of 15f and g)			88	67
i. Percent Paid (15c divided by 15f times 100)			77.77%	86%

* If you are claiming electronic copies, go to line 16 on page 3. If you are not claiming electronic copies, skip to line 17 on page 3.

16. Electronic Copy Circulation

	Average No. Copies Each Issue During Preceding 12 Months	No. Copies of Single Issue Published Nearest to Filing Date
a. Paid Electronic Copies ▶		
b. Total Paid Print Copies (Line 15c) + Paid Electronic Copies (Line 16a) ▶		
c. Total Print Distribution (Line 15f) + Paid Electronic Copies (Line 16a) ▶		
d. Percent Paid (Both Print & Electronic Copies) (16b divided by 16c × 100) ▶		

☒ I certify that 50% of all my distributed copies (electronic and print) are paid above a nominal price.

17. Publication of Statement of Ownership
☒ If the publication is a general publication, publication of this statement is required. Will be printed
in the DECEMBER 2022 issue of this publication. ☐ Publication not required.

18. Signature and Title of Editor, Publisher, Business Manager, or Owner

Malathi Samayan - Distribution Controller   *Malathi Samayan*   Date 9/18/2022

I certify that all information furnished on this form is true and complete. I understand that anyone who furnishes false or misleading information on this form or who omits material or information requested on the form may be subject to criminal sanctions (including fines and imprisonment) and/or civil sanctions (including civil penalties).

PS Form **3526**, July 2014 (Page 3 of 4) PRIVACY NOTICE: See our privacy policy on www.usps.com

Printed and bound by CPI Group (UK) Ltd, Croydon, CR0 4YY

03/10/2024

01040467-0017